Golf Flex

Golf Flex

The Complete Workout

10 MINUTES A DAY TO BETTER PLAY

FLEXIBILITY AND STRENGTH
CONDITIONING FOR BETTER GOLF

Paul Frediani

A GetFitNow.com Book

HATHERLEIGH PRESS

New York • London

Golf Flex: The Complete Workout
A GETFITNOW.com Book

Hatherleigh Press/GETFITNOW.com Books
An Affiliate of W.W. Norton & Company, Inc.
5-22 46th Avenue, Suite 200
Long Island City, NY 11101
1-800-367-2550
Visit our website: www.getfitnow.com

Disclaimer:
Before beginning any exercise program consult your physician. The author and publisher of this book and workout disclaim any liability, personal or professional, resulting from the misapplication of any of the training procedures described in this publication.

All GETFITNOW.com titles are available for bulk purchase, special promotions, and premiums. For more information, please contact the manager of our Special Sales Department at 1-800-528-2550.

Library of Congress Cataloging-in-Publication Data
Frediani, Paul, 1952-
  Golf flex : the complete workout / Paul Frediani.
     p. cm.
  "A Getfitnow.com book."
  ISBN 1-57826-155-4
  1. Golf--Training. 2. Stretching exercises. I. Title.
  GV979.E9F74 2005
  613.7'11--dc22
                          2005006625

Cover design by Lisa Fyfe and Phillip Mondestin
Text design by Deborah Miller

Principle photography by Peter Field Peck
Printed in Canada on acid-free paper
10 9 8 7 6 5 4 3

Additional photography copyright of Digital Stock,
A division of Corbis Corporation.

Quotations from golf pros courtesy of www.PGA.com, the official web site of The PGA of America.

Acknowledgments

A big thanks to:

Matt Bloom, for getting the ball rolling

Tracy Tumminello, for her patience, encouragement, and editing talent

and Renee Meier, my love and guardian angel.

A special thanks to the following leaders in the fitness industry who are my friends, educators, and motivators, without whose passion and support this would not be possible: Annette Lang, Dos Condon, Bob Esquerre, and Rocco Greco.

Special thanks to my publishers Andrew Flach and Kevin Moran, my editor Andrea Au, assistant editor Alyssa Smith, and photographer Peter Peck. All made working on Golf Flex a pleasure.

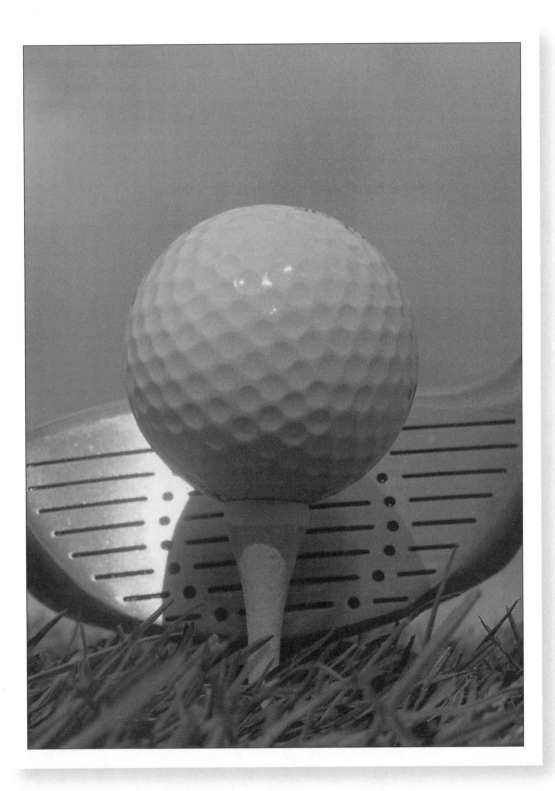

Contents

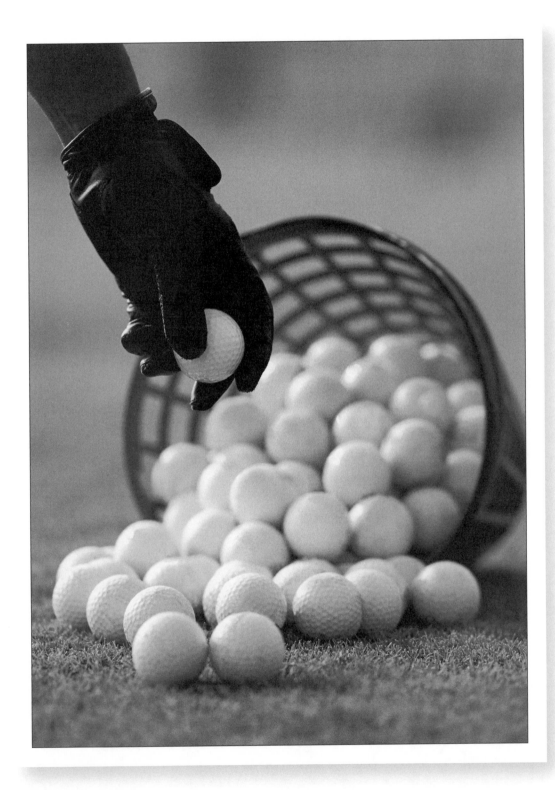

Introduction

WELCOME TO THE NEW AND UPDATED *GOLF FLEX!* If you're new to Golf Flex, this is the first step to improve your flexibility, strength, and fitness to enhance your golf game. If you've a returning reader, welcome back. My name is Paul Frediani and I am a fitness advisor and have been a personal trainer for over 12 years.

I have seen numerous fads in the fitness industry come and go. What is considered the best exercise one year can be disproven the next. Staying informed of current exercise science is difficult not only for the layperson but also for fitness professional.

The better condition you are in, if you are a weekend warrior or a competitive athlete, will determine how quickly you can improve your skills. This will also reduce your risk of sports related injuries. Physical conditioning and technical skill conditioning are two different elements for the development of golf and should be addressed separately. The strongest man in the world is not the one who can hit skillfully hit the longest drive nor can the most skilled of golfers reach their peak potential if they are not in the best physical condition. *Golf Flex* is focused on getting you in your top physical condition. It does not address the high levels of technical skills required for playing golf. Skill and technique training requires you to work with your golf pro.

Here is the latest on golfer's flexibility and functional strength training using the fitness ball. I've cut through all the fitness jargon to bring you what you need to know in its simplest form, and have tried to dispel some preconceived myths regarding stretching and strength training.

The original *Golf Flex* focused on flexibility and pre-game warm-up, and was easy for the everyday golfer to incorporate. In the same style, I will keep the strength programs applicable and to the point. In my experience, complex fitness programs don't work because they confuse and dishearten exercisers, in addition to being time consuming and boring. No exercise program will help your game or your fitness if it's not being followed. I'll take a fast, fun, and effective exercise program over a long, laborious, and tedious one anytime!

The new *Golf Flex* Strength Training Fitness Program is easy to follow, simple, quick, and enjoyable. The key we will focus upon for increased conditioning and flexibility is above all, consistency. We're all interested in maintaining independence in our lives. We all want to be healthy, mobile, and fit. Staying in shape and being flexible and strong will not only improve your golf, but your day-to-day life. How counterproductive to your health would it be if just trying to find the time in your day to workout causes you stress? For some just the thought of exercising for 1 or 1-1/2 hours is enough to defeat them. Time constraints are a prime reason people don't exercise. If looking forward to your present exercise program feels like looking forward to a root canal, then I think my strength program is for you. Most everyone can find 30 minutes a few times a week to workout. As you will see, exercising on a ball is fun, gets you results, and you don't need to be a PhD to follow the programs. You also don't need a gym membership, personal trainer, or expensive equipment. All you need is a few dumbbells and an exercise ball and you're ready to go!

Part I:
Golf: An Athletic Event Or Recreational Pasttime?

THERE WAS A TIME NOT TOO LONG AGO WHERE THE AMOUNT OF WEIGHT a golfer lifted depended on whether it was a pint or a rocks glass. Flexibility was the ability to tie your shoes without groaning. Cardiovascular fitness meant walking instead of taking a cart. Aah! The good old days!

In every sport that exists today, athletes have improved performance. Today's athletes are physically superior to athletes of the past. They run faster, jump higher, and perform longer. World records constantly are being set. The pitchers in the World Series are in their 40s. The modern athlete has taken huge steps past those in the 60's not because of greater skills but the advantage of today's modern training techniques and a greater understanding of exercise physiology. Not only are athletes playing at a heightened level; they achieve and maintain their highest level of performance at the latter part of their career. Elite golfers play longer and stronger because their conditioning programs keep them injury-free and at a high level of fitness.

Golfers pour money into the billon-dollar golf industry for the latest pieces of equipment; balls that fly further or clubs with bigger sweet spots. Yet despite technological advances in equipment, average golf scores have not improved over the years.

Dr. Bob Rotella, author of *Golf of Your Dreams*, said "15 years ago the average amateur male golfer handicap was 16.5, the average female 29." These remain the same today. So, shall we continue to invest in the latest piece of equipment on the market, hoping it will improve your game, or shall you invest in the most valuable piece of equipment you possess: your body?

Golf is an athlete's game. According to Dr. Donald Chu, a fitness expert, "the energy of hitting a golf ball 300 yards is the same as hitting a baseball 300 feet. A 10 handicap golfer will take about 50 hard swings per game, 50-75 more in practice." That's a lot of energy output! A golfer also picks-up 1/3 of their body weight 30 to 40 times per game and walks thousands of yards.

Golfers, like other athletes, must maintain good flexibility. Pick up any golfers' magazine or journal and they will be filled with advice, including tips for one's swing like "keep loose," "rotate more," "strong but supple," "relaxed." What they fail to do is tell you how to get there! Staying flexible may seem like an uphill battle, but improvements can be made in as little as 10 minutes a day. A daily 8 to 10 minute static stretching routine does much more than stretching one time, one hour a week. As we age, our joints and muscles naturally get tighter, and this has a terrible effect on our swing and our lower back. Not only will stretching improve your game, it will also help you avoid injuries.

According to the American Academy of Orthopedic Surgeons, anywhere from 45% to 80% of golfers have lower back pain. In 1991 there were 7,000 reported golf injuries, and in 1998, 14,000. The American Academy of Orthopedic Surgeons recommends warm-up and stretching before playing to avoid injury. If we choose to ignore their advice, we can expect to be a number in their golf injury statistics sheet.

Although not many of us are in Tiger's league, we can still benefit from the training used by elite athletes. Regardless of one's age or playing ability, stretching, proper warm-ups, and strength training will keep you healthy and on the course.

Part II:
Flexology: The Importance Of
Golf Flex, Or, Why Stretch?

STRETCHING IS OFTEN MISUNDERSTOOD AND EVEN MORE OFTEN poorly performed. There are several stretching methods and if you ask different fitness experts you'll get different opinions on which are the best and at what time to do them. To start understanding this complex subject, you should start with the terms flexibility, mobility, and warming up. All are often used interchangeably and sometimes poorly preformed. I will try and make some sense of them. The one benefit about stretching we do know for sure is that we need to stretch because as we get older we will get tighter and our range of motion (ROM) becomes limited.

Stretching does not simply warm up your muscles, but over a period of time, increases the flexibility of the muscles themselves. Flexion is defined as an act of bending or being bent without breaking. Good flexibility for golfers implies having the proper ROM at all the joints and muscles needed so as to not hinder a smooth swing. When we stretch, we are lengthening the belly of the muscle as well as the fascia surrounding the muscle. When muscles are lengthened they are relaxed and retain their optimum range of motion. Imagine your golf swing if you took away 10% ROM of your back swing and 10% ROM of your follow through, it would reduce the length of your drives.

If you added 10% in your take away and 10% in your follow through you would increase the length of your drives. Maintaining or increasing flexibility to your muscles will give your swing the fullest range of motion and thus better golf performance and distance. On the other hand, being inflexible creates poor posture and a tight swing, and an increased risk of joint overuse injuries and makes for poor swing mechanics.

Mobility deals with your body's joints and ligaments. Tendons attach muscles to bones, and ligaments attach bones to bones. We don't stretch ligaments, we increase joint mobility by gentle and small rocking movements. These movements should never be forceful and should always follow the normal direction of the joint movement. Your joint mobility should be balanced with your joint stability to create a smooth swing. Too loose of a joint and you won't have proper control, and too tight of a joint and your swing won't have power behind it. It is easy to mistake joint mobility with muscular flexibility because it's possible to have good muscular flexibility but poor joint mobility or visa versa. It is also possible to have ideal mobility in one joint and a lack on it in another. This of course can create havoc when trying to develop a consistent swing. Improving your golf swing requires a good range of motion, or a combination of flexibility, stability, and joint mobility.

How and when we warm up and stretch is important. The conventional method used to be: warming up your core temperature with light cardio for 8 to 10 minutes, then statically stretching. This really didn't make any sense, because by the end of stretching, your core temperature would have returned to where it was before you began your cardio. So what would the point be in the warm-up? Shouldn't the point of warming-up be preparation for playing not for stretching? Confusing? You bet.

More so the latest research shows that slow static stretching before exercise does not decrease the risk of injury or increase sports performance. Why? Well, consider this. How does your body feel after a long slow static stretching session? Great, right? You feel so relaxed that you could easily take a nap. That's also exactly how it makes your muscles feel: dormant. Do you want dormant muscles before you pick up your club and demand your body to swing it over 100 miles per hour? How would your body react feel if I entered your bedroom at 5 a.m., woke you up by playing reveille on my bugle and forced you to run a mile? A little shocking to your system?

Dynamic stretching is how you should prepare yourself for your golf game. Static stretching involves holding a stretch for 20 seconds and longer, much like yoga. With dynamic stretching, you move you in and out of the stretch for a brief second, resembling calisthenics. You will be warming up and increasing your body temperature, get-

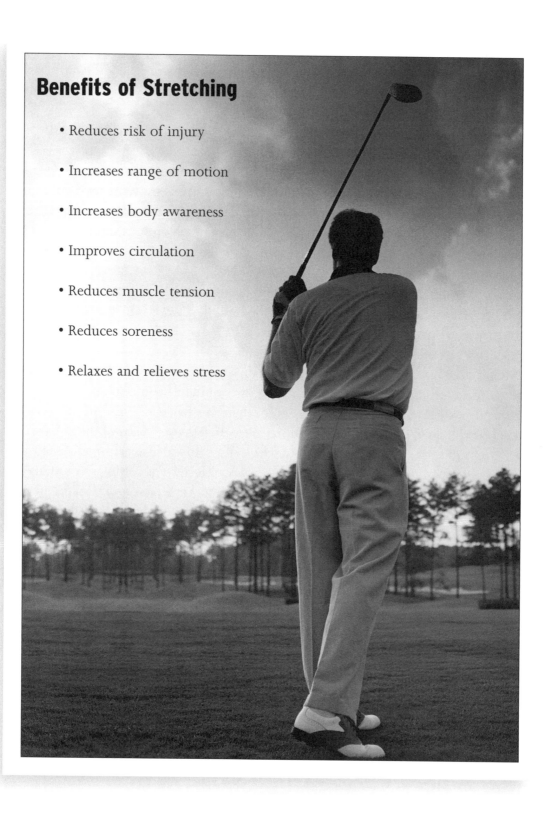

Benefits of Stretching

- Reduces risk of injury

- Increases range of motion

- Increases body awareness

- Improves circulation

- Reduces muscle tension

- Reduces soreness

- Relaxes and relieves stress

ting an uptake in your cardio and blood to your muscles, increasing body awareness and balance, and lubing up your joints. This is how you prepare your body for the task at hand and not waste 3 holes getting warmed up when you can be ready to play on the first hole.

That's not to say static stretching is bad. Static stretching is still great! Ask David Duval, Jesper Parnevik, Annika Sorenstam, and Se Ri Pak why they do yoga. However, static stretching is what you want to do after your game to cool down and help remove lactic acid (a byproduct from your muscles). Or during the week, to increase your range of motion and joint mobility, especially targeting the muscle groups that are tight. An exception to this is if you have any type of joint degeneration. You should avoid static stretching of that specific joint. Use instead dynamic stretching because it will increase blood flow and nutrients to the diseased joint.

Keep in mind that not everyone is in need of stretching. Wow! Did I say that? You'd think I didn't want to sell my book? It's true. Some fitness experts forget to tell you that some of you are hyper flexible or hyper mobile. (Women, are you listening?) This condition can place the health of your joints in jeopardy and affect your golf performance. You don't need to stretch if you're over-flexible. In any yoga class you'll see many more women there are than men. Why is that? Because women for the most part are more flexible than men. In the weight lifting room, there are twice as many men as women. That's because men, on average, have more muscular strength than women. A person, when given the choice, will always take the path of least resistance, as opposed to need. If your body was a guitar and you wanted it to play sweetly, your strings would have to be tuned at the correct tension. If some of your strings were loose you wouldn't loosen them more, you would tighten them. If you're hyper flexible or hyper-mobile what you need is more stability and strength training. The pre-game dynamic warm-up should still be what you do before your game. You should avoid slow static stretches and spend more time with strengthening and stabilization exercises.

Stretching Myths

Myth 1—It's too time-consuming. There's no way I can fit it in my busy schedule.

You do not need to take time out from your day to stretch. You can start a flexibility program before you even get out of bed, while working in the office, or even in the car.

Myth 2—Flexibility training is for professional athletes only. It is much too complex to do alone. I would have to hire a personal trainer and spend a fortune.

Golf Flex is as easy as one, two, three. Complex fitness programs just don't work. If you have read this far, you're smart enough to follow this program. Save your money to buy new clubs.

Myth 3—I will never be flexible.

You will never be flexible if you don't stretch. It may be true that you'll never do splits, but short of major injuries, you can significantly improve your range of motion. The aging process naturally shortens and tightens your muscles. Flexibility training can help reverse that process.

Myth 4—I don't need to stretch everyday. I just stretch well once a week before I play.

Stretching once a week will do this for you—absolutely nothing. To increase your range of motion or improve flexibility, you need to stretch ten minutes a day. Consistency is the key.

Myth 5—Stretching is so boring.

Think about adding 20 to 40 yards to your drive. Boring? I think not. Professional golfers are adding that much yardage to their game simply because they have discovered the indisputable benefits of stretching. Lack of flexibility can make your golf swing short and narrow, reducing distance on your drive. So think about that when you start to yawn. What can be more boring than sitting home tending to your injuries? Reduce flexibility and you will increase your potential for serious injury.

Myth 6–I am too old to stretch.

It's never too late to begin a flexibility program. There is no better time than right now! If you want to be successful, avoid injuries, and have the satisfaction of a better game, stretching is the key. What are you waiting for? There are people running marathons in their 70s and 80s. Today's 70s were Yesterday's 50s. Let's get busy! Let's stay active! Just a few minutes a day and you will see how much more limber you feel after only a few weeks.

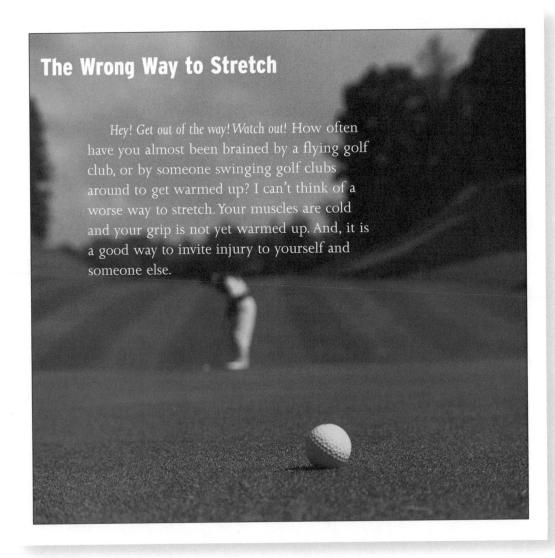

The Wrong Way to Stretch

Hey! Get out of the way! Watch out! How often have you almost been brained by a flying golf club, or by someone swinging golf clubs around to get warmed up? I can't think of a worse way to stretch. Your muscles are cold and your grip is not yet warmed up. And, it is a good way to invite injury to yourself and someone else.

Improving Your Range Of Motion

"Spend 5 to 7 minutes stretching and mentally preparing how you want to play."

—John Stacey, PGA Pro

Stretching can be a daily part of your life because you can incorporate it in every part of your routine. It will become as natural as bushing your teeth. Please remember that stretching is not a competition! You won't get flexible in a day. One sure way to get injured is to overstretch (the too far too fast symptom). This was why doctors offices were full of patients injured from yoga when yoga hit the mainstream. It wasn't the dangers of yoga; it was the individual's own aggressive approach.

Your daily living activities can hinder and create tightness and poor posture. Some of the simplest everyday tasks can, after a period of time, destroy your body. Here are a few: carrying a bag slung over your shoulder, carrying that wallet in your back pocket, hunching over your desk at work, sitting for prolonged periods with your legs crossed, high heels, prolonged standing with weight shifted on one leg, poor choice of exercises, sedentary lifestyle, and lack of exercise. The list can go on and on. These may seem small, but if drops of water drip on a rock for a long enough period of time the drops will shape the rock. What may seem small and inconsequential daily living activates are very important for you to become alert to. Drop by drop you may be creating poor posture. The first step in correcting them is to become aware of these poor habits and to be alert to your posture. Simply by improving your posture will give you an opportunity to achieve your full potential.

Rotational Posture Test

Try this test. Sit on a chair with poor posture. Slumped with your head sticking forward. Now cross your arms across your chest and turn your torso to look behind you. Keep in mind the distance you've rotated. Now sit up straight, chest high, shoulder back and turn again. How much more rotation did you achieve? Amazing huh?

Water, water, water. How much do you drink? Do you know that most of us walk around in a dehydrated state? A great portion of people that complain of back pain are only dehydrated and can solve their problems by just drinking the proper amount of water. The disc that separates our vertebrae contains 85% to 90% water, and the loss of water in the disk makes them less effective as shock absorbers and results in disc degeneration. Many of the world's leading fitness experts believe you should drink half your body weight in ounces of water. (If you weighed 180 pounds, you should be drinking 90 ounces of water per day.) I have personally witnessed many of my clients increase their flexibility and reduce their back pain within just one week of increasing water consumption.

Do not wait to drink until your thirsty. At that point, its already too late and you are well on your way to being dehydrated. As we get older, it is even more important to monitor how much we drink because the mechanism that tells us we are thirsty becomes dormant. Remember that caffeine, diet sodas, and alcohol do not count as they actually dehydrate you.

The Science of *Golf Flex*

Power is force produced over a distance per unit of time. In golf, power is the result of a total body as a chainlink summation of coordinated movements. If any of these three elements can be increased—force exerted, speed (unit of time at the head of the club during the downswing), or range of motion (flexibility)—the result will be a longer drive.

Part III:
Flexology Assessments

-*"The most important aspect of a good golf swing is the stretch of the muscles."*

—David Glenz, PGA Pro

THE FOLLOWING AREAS OF THE BODY ARE IMPORTANT to the overall flexibility program for golfers. Let's address these areas and how they relate to your golf swing. The swing is a complex action which uses many muscle groups together in a synchronized chain of events. The body during the golf swing moves in integration, not isolation. The following muscle groups work in unison to give you a fluid swing.

The assessments are of the normal ranges of motion. Lack of these can be hindering your full potential. Make a note of your assessments and then use the exercises listed to help improve them. Retest yourself every 30 days.

Neck While standing at address, your neck is in flexion and there is undo stress on the back of your neck. Warming up your neck with head rolls is a great way to prepare for the ball impact and rotation of the torso.

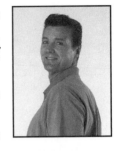

The Fault Reduced neck rotation makes it hard to keep your eye on the ball during the swing.

Assessment You should be able to turn your head so that your chin is directly over the shoulder, or approximately 45 degrees.

Flexibility Solution Yes and No stretches done with static holds of 10 to 20 seconds. You can give this stretch assistance by adding light pressure from your hand.

Strength Solution Give your head gentle resistance with your hand when doing the Yes and Nos.

Upper Back and Shoulders Increasing flexibility in the upper back and shoulders will assist in providing greater rotation and range of motion in both your back swing and your follow through. Increasing strength here will result in more speed and power.

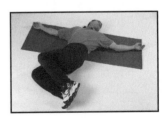

The Fault Tight internal rotation of the your left arm or tight external rotation of your left shoulder reduces the range of your take away. Tight external rotation of your right arm or tight internal rotation of your right shoulder reduces the range of your follow through.

Assessment Place one hand behind your head and touch the top of the opposite shoulder blade. At the same time, place the opposing hand behind your back and touch the bottom of its opposite shoulder blade. If your hands are more than one hand width distance apart you're too tight. As pictured, the model's hands should touch the lines.

Flexibility Solution Back Scratches, Back Stretchers, Bye-Byes, Toweling Off, and static holds of 15-20 seconds

Strength Solution Shoulder Set, One Arm Row

Lower Back and Trunk This is definitely the most crucial of areas to keep flexible, strong, and stable. The golf swing relies heavily on your back for stabilization and rotation. This is the most commonly injured and strained area for both PGA and amateur golfers. The lower back and your trunk are the

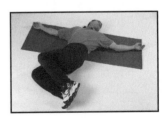

center of your power drive. Did you know that every time you bend over to pick up a ball, you lift half of your body weight?

The Fault Less trunk rotation will limit your shoulder turning ability and create a faulty swing and potential injury in the lower back

The Assessment Lie on your back, extend your arms out to the sides, and then bend your knees and fold them over to one side, allowing your knees to lie on the floor. The back of your opposite shoulder should stay in contact with the ground.

Flexibility Solution At the Office, Helicopters, Peach Pickers, Corkscrews, In Bed, Hamstrings

Strength Solution Core sets, Superman, Lois Lane, Swimmer

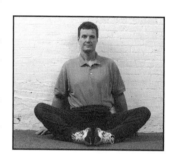

Inner/Outer Hips If you want to generate more power and have monster drives, you've got to be able to crisply transfer your weight. All sports require hip-to-shoulder rotation, from boxing to swimming. If you cannot rotate your hips, you cannot deliver power to your upper body and shoulders from your legs.

The Fault You are unable to transfer weight or stabilize the lower extremities.

Assessment Sit on the floor with your back to a wall. Be sure your lower back is touching the wall. Bring your feet together and move them toward your groin. You knees should be at a 45-degree angle.

Flexibility Solution Putting on Socks and Shoes, At the Office, Tinkerbell, Butterfly, Corkscrew, Indian Sits, and Inner Thigh

Strength Solution Scissors, Inner Thigh Lift

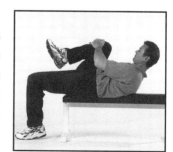

Hip Flexor/Quad Quads, the big muscles at the fronts of your legs, are responsible for knee extensions. The hip flexor is responsible for the flexion of your hip. This muscle runs from the front of the hip to the lumbar region. A tight hip flexor muscle pulls on the lower back and is often a culprit of lower back pain.

The Fault Tight hip flexors create stress on the lower back. Tight quads (complete)

Assessment Lie on your back with your hips on the edge on a bench. Take one knee and bring it toward your chest. Observe the opposite leg. The thigh should be parallel to the floor with the knee at a 90-degree angle.

Flexibility Solution Thigh Stretch on Exercise Ball, Putting on Sock and Shoes, Quadriceps Stretch

Strength Solution Lunge and Squat sets.

Hamstrings Hamstrings are a notoriously tight muscle group, especially for those with sedentary jobs. Tight hamstrings can cause havoc on your posture and problems with the lower back.

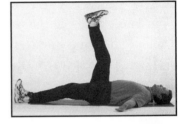

The Fault You are unable to get into or properly hold good posture during set-up.

Assessment Lie on your back on the floor. Lift one leg up and keep the opposite leg on the floor. Anything less than a 90-degree angle of the lifted leg mean you have tight hamstrings.

Flexibility Solution Hamstring Stretch, Hamstring Stretch on Exercise Ball, Toweling Off.

Strength Solution Hamstring Curls, Hip Extensions on Exercise Ball.

Mechanics of the Golf Swing

Let's take a look at the mechanics of a golf swing and how improving your flexibility can create more power in your drive. The golf swing is a complex motion, requiring the use of many joints in your body. The more joints incorporated in any movement, whether it be golf, baseball, football, basketball, or another activity, the more torque and power your body can create in the movement.

You begin the golf swing as you address the ball with your ankles and knees slightly flexed. The leg, butt, and back muscles are engaged. The abdominal muscles are tight to protect the lower back, and the neck is flexed forward.

The right hip initiates the backswing as you shift your weight to your right foot. Rotation begins with your knees and your left hip rotates forward. The right side of your waist turns your torso as your shoulder muscles pull the club back. The rotator cuffs stabilize the shoulder girdle, and your elbow and wrist joints are both flexed. This action is reversed during the downswing and follow through.

By increasing the range of motion in all your joints and surrounding muscles, and by increasing the strength in your abdominal muscles you are better able to deliver the power of your legs and hips to your upper torso and shoulders and thus more horsepower in your swing.

Part IV:
The *Golf Flex* Pre-Game Warm-Up

THESE ARE 19 DYNAMIC STRETCHING MOVEMENTS for total your pre-game warm-up. This warm up should take you 8 to 12 minutes, total, to complete. Move in and out of the stretch point without a prolonged hold, at a one count (one-one thousand) at the stretch point. Stay on each stretch roughly 30 seconds. By the end of the warm-up you should have a slight elevation of your heart rate and a slight dampness on your forehead. It will take only a few times to memorize the 19 movements. Don't worry if you forget a few of the stretches. This isn't an exact science, and the point is to get the benefits of warming-up. After a few times you will be able to go through them all with no problem.

Before you begin, some important points to remember:

1. Always remember to breathe. Don't hold your breath.
2. Maintain good posture, which opens the pathways for creating good movement patterns.
3. The movements are brisk. They never bounce or jerk.
4. Commit to being consistent. Consistently doing an abbreviated 5-minute warm-up is better than nothing.
5. Pain is not gain. If it's painful, it isn't right.
6. Focus on your body: mindless movements achieve mindless results.
7. Don't over do it. Stretching is not a race or competition.
8. Be sure you consult with your doctor before beginning this or any flexibility program.
9. Listen to what your body is telling you, it's your best teacher.
10. Smile, it keeps your face relaxed and body loose. And remember to breathe. Like Tom Sutter said, "A tight mind is a tight body".

Breathing

If you want to stay loose and flexible, you have to breathe. I know what you're thinking: "I don't need to learn how to breathe, I've been doing it all my life." You are right, but chances are you're not breathing correctly. Think about it, of food, water, and breath, which do you require above all? Even so, I know that most people breathe incorrectly.

Breath is life, and breathing properly will give you more vitality, energy, focus, and relaxation. All of these elements you need in golf to stay in the "zone". Did you know that in a 4 hour round of golf, the actual time spent hitting the ball is four minutes? That means you have plenty of time to think about your next shot, which gives you lots of time to get mentally tight or stressed between shots. Staying connected and breathing properly between swings will help you stay loose.

If you want to see a perfect example of breathing, watch a baby breathe. They have no physical obstacles like a tense stomach, inflexible rib cage, poor posture, mental stress, tension; they only have purely natural, uninhibited breathing. A relaxed body and perfect breath is the door to good performance.

There are 3 levels of breathing: diaphragmatic, intercostals, and clavicular. The ideal breath combines all three types.

During Diaphragmatic breathing, the breath is drawn in, the diaphragm is lowered, and the abdominal region swells. Good breath control starts here.

Intercostal breathing raises the chest and the thoracic ribs. It's quite common for athletes to breathe this way, but it takes more effort and allows less air to enter.

If you raise your shoulders and collarbone while inhaling, this is clavicular breathing. Only the upper lungs are fully functional.

A complete and full breath begins at the diaphragm. It swells the abdominals, then the ribs, and the chest, all naturally allowing the lungs to completely fill up as high as the collarbones.

The average rate of breath is 12 to 14 times a minute, but the actual optimal healthy rate is only 6 breaths per minute. If you're breathing 12 to 14 times per minute, you are in a slight state of hyperventilation. Taking these quick shallow breaths reduces the level of carbon dioxide in your body which constricts your arteries and reduces the flow of blood through the body. The lack of oxygen switches on the sympathetic nervous system (fight or flight reflex) and makes us tense and anxious. Is that how you want to feel in a tight situation?

The 3 Part Breath Exercise

Part One

Lay on your back, place your hand on your belly with your thumb above bellybutton and your other four fingers below. Breathe in and allow your belly to expand under your hand. Take five breaths slowly in at a 5 count, exhaling also at a 5 count.

Part Two

Place your other hand on your lower ribs. Breathe in and first feel the lower belly expand and then allow and feel the ribs expand. Take five breaths slowly in at a 5 count, exhaling at a 5 count.

Part Three

Breathe in and build your breath, filling first your belly then your ribs. Allow the top of the chest to fill. This process should begin slowly, allowing each section time to fill. Do not force the breath, this should take place naturally. Take five breaths slowly in at a 5 count, exhaling at a 5 count

Repeat this process ten times. As you become more comfortable with the process, increase the 2 count by two. Always breathe through your nose.

The Golf Flex 10 Minutes a Day Pre-Game Warm-Up Program

1. Yes and Nos
2. Shoulder Rolls
3. Back Scratchers
4. Back Stretcher
5. Tree Hugger
6. Rooster Crow
7. Bye-Byes
8. Peach Pickers
9. Willow Tree
10. Wrist Roll with Finger Spreader
11. Forearm Flex and Stretch
12. Helicopters
13. Hula Hoops
14. Hamstrings
15. Quadriceps
16. Calves & Achilles
17. Knee and Ankle Roll
18. Inner Thigh
19. Hay Balers

Did you know that tightness is often a sign of muscular weakness? Flexibility and strength training go hand in hand. Identify your weakness and improve your strength.

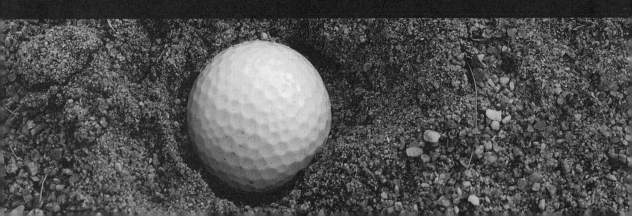

1. Yes and No

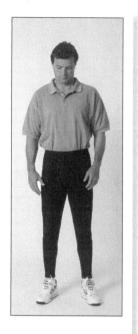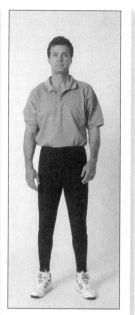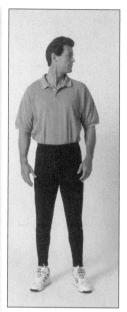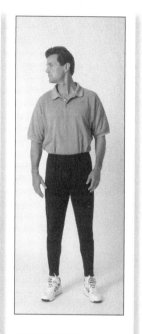

Nod your head "Yes" by bringing your chin to your chest, then back up to the neutral position. Start the "No" movement by facing forward, turning your head slowly to the left until your chin is over your left shoulder, then slowly to the right until your chin is over the right shoulder. Neck exercises should be done gently. Repeat this exercise eight times.

Muscles used: Neck muscles.

Result: Prepares and warms up the neck for shoulder rotation and the impact of hitting the ball.

Tip: Add half moon rolls, which are chin rolls from one shoulder to the chest to the other shoulder. Be careful not to extend the neck backward.

2. Shoulder Rolls

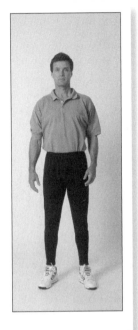 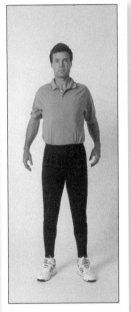 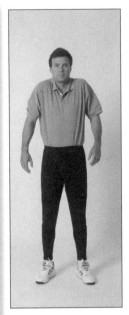 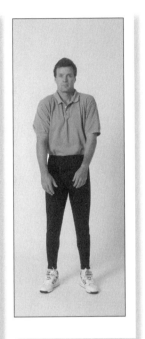

Lift your shoulders to your ears—forward, down, back, and up. Reverse directions, and repeat the motion eight times both ways.

Muscles used: Shoulder muscles.

Result: Warms up the shoulders and prepares the neck for the impact of the swing.

Tip: Great stretch to relieve neck and shoulder tension.

3. Back Scratchers

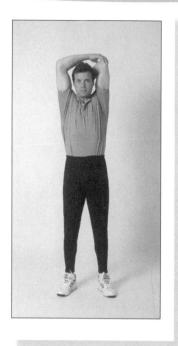 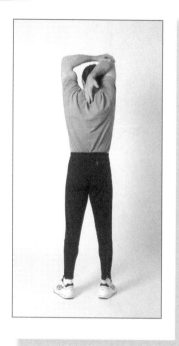 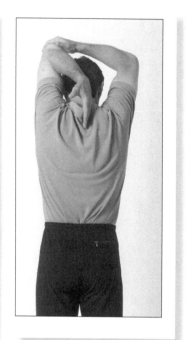

Reach one elbow up toward the ceiling and your hand behind your neck and toward the opposite shoulder. With the other hand, assist the stretch by gently pulling back on the elbow. Repeat eight times on both sides.

Muscles used: Backs of arms, shoulders, and back muscles.

Result: Improves backswing, downswing, impact, and follow through.

Tip: Bend at the waist to increase the stretch.

4. Back Stretcher

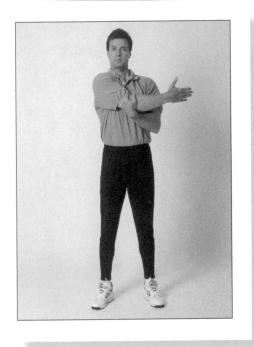 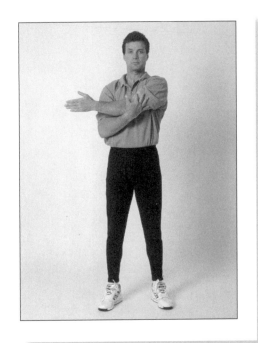

Keeping your shoulders down, stretch your right arm across your chest, and gently pull your right arm towards you with your left hand. You can add more intensity by turning your torso. Switch arms and repeat eight times on both sides.

Muscles used: Upper back, arms, and shoulder muscles.

Result: Improves backswing and follow through.

Tip: Keep your shoulders down and away from the ears.

5. Tree Hugger

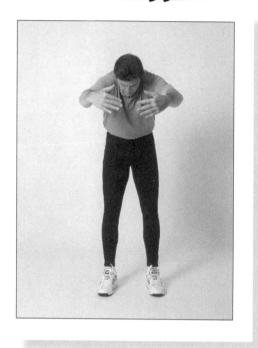 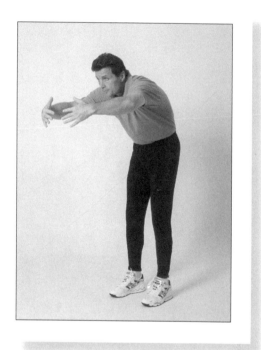

With your feet shoulder width apart, pretend you're wrapping your arms around a big tree. Keep your chin to your chest as you contract your stomach muscles. You will feel this stretch from your tailbone to the top of your head. Repeat ten times.

Muscles used: Full back and spine stretch.

Result: Helps backswing, downswing, and impact.

Tip: Be sure to keep your abdominal muscles tight.

6. Rooster Crows

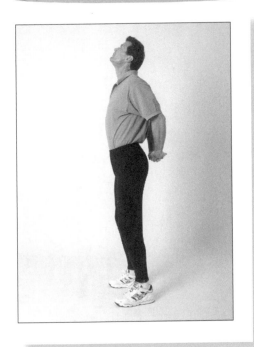 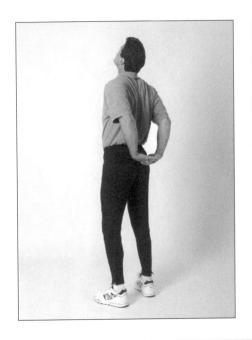

Interlace your fingers behind your back. Squeeze your shoulder blades together as you stick our your chest, pressing your hands backward. Look up toward the ceiling, contract your butt, and stretch the front of your shoulders and chest. You want to keep your chest open to achieve a greater range of motion in both your back and forward swings. Combine wit the Tree Hugger stretch, and repeat ten times.

Muscles used: Chest, front of shoulders, and upper back muscles.

Result: Improves backswing and follow through.

Tip: A slight arch in the lower back will increase this stretch. When stretching, remember your ears and shoulders are mortal enemies. Keep your shoulders down!

7. Bye-Byes

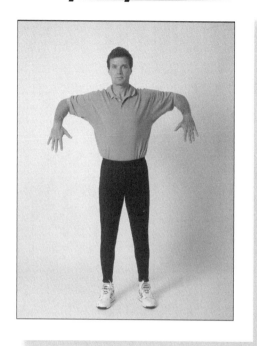 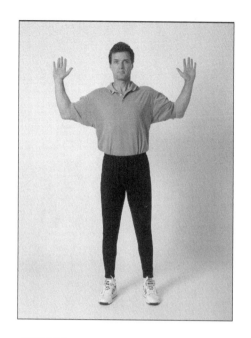

With your arms out to the sides, bend your forearms up from the elbows 90 degrees with your palms facing forward. Then, rotate your forearms, pressing your palms down. Repeat eight times.

Muscles used: Rotator Cuffs.

Result: Benefits the backswing, downswing, impact, and follow through.

Tip: Keep your shoulders stable and only rotate the arms. Work smoothly and slowly.

8. Peach Pickers

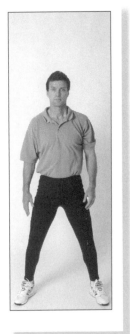 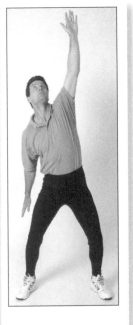 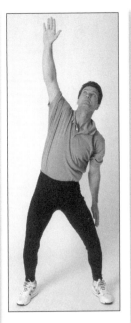 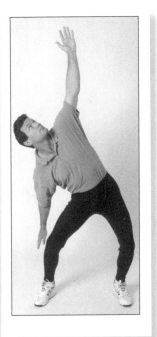

With your feet shoulder width apart and your knees slightly bent, keep your stomach tight as you reach one hand toward the ceiling and the other toward the floor. Stretch your waist and shoulders as you alternate hands. Repeat the motion eight times. Advanced–For a more intense stretch, reach further and bend more from the waist.

Muscles used: Waist and shoulder muscles.

Result: Improves backswing, downswing, and follow through.

Tip: Deepen your knees by bending and reaching laterally to increase your stretch.

9. Willow Tree

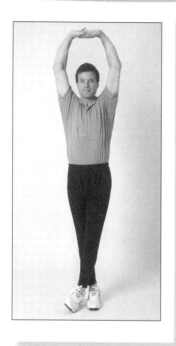 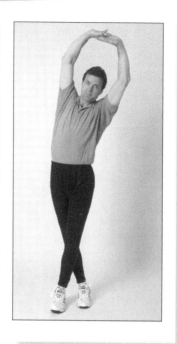 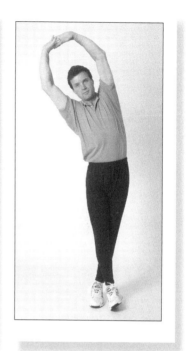

Cross your feet, interlace your fingers, and reach the palms of your hands toward the ceiling. Advanced–Bend from the torso from side to side four times. Switch feet position and repeat.

Muscles used: Forearms, arms, fingers, shoulders, waist, hips, and legs.

Result: Improves address, backswing, downswing, and prepares the upper body for impact with the ball.

Tip: Keep your abdominal muscles contracted and your butt tight.

10. Wrist Roll with Finger Spreader

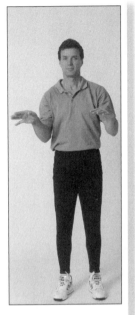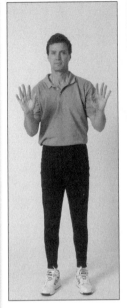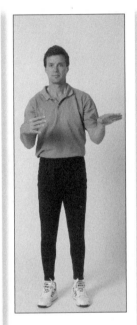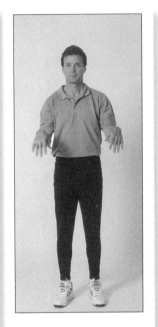

With your fingers loose, roll your wrists clockwise, then counter-clockwise five times.

Advanced: Press the tips of your fingers together as you separate your palms, stretching your fingers apart.

Muscles used: Hand and wrist muscles.

Result: Helps address and prepares the hands and wrists for impact with the ball.

Tip: If needed, repeat during play to help alleviate post-game soreness.

11. Forearm Flex and Stretch

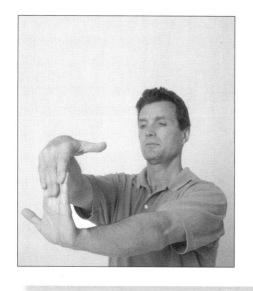
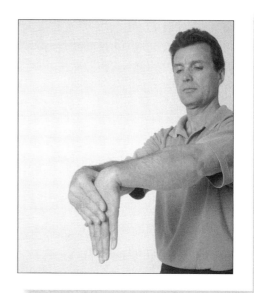

With one arm extended in front of you, gently press your fingers down with your opposite hand, palms inward. Repeat the motion pulling your fingers back with your palms facing outward. Perform this stretch five times on each hand.

Muscles used: Forearm muscles.

Result: Improves address and prepares the forearms for impact with the ball.

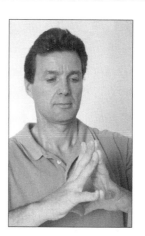

Tip: This stretch, in combination with strengthening exercises, will help prevent Golfers' Elbow.

12. Helicopters

Stand with your feet shoulder width apart and your arms extended out to the sides. Keep your face and hips forward as you rotate your torso to the left and right, keeping your arms straight.

Advanced: Twist your torso as you reach your right hand to your left pocket and your left hand to your right pocket. This stretch is excellent for torso rotation. Switch sides and repeat ten times.

Muscles used: Waist and torso muscles.

Result: Improves your backswing, downswing, and follow through.

Tip: Start slowly and keep your face forward, increasing your rotation as you progress. Be sure your abdominal muscles are tight and your knees bent.

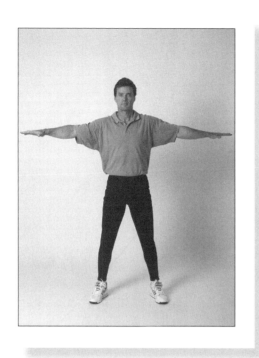 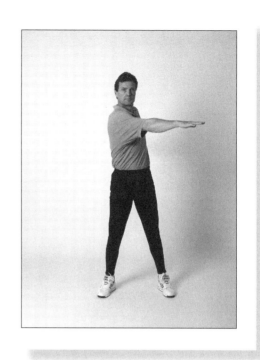

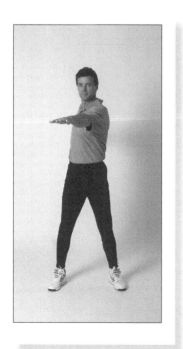 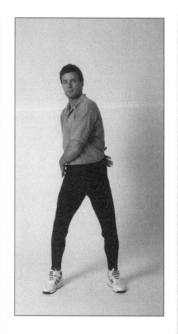 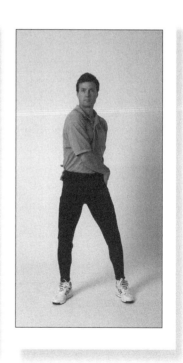

13. Hula Hoops

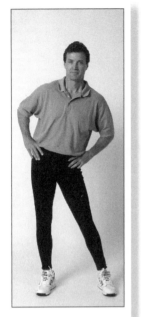 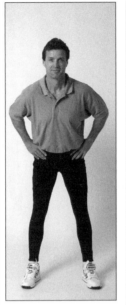 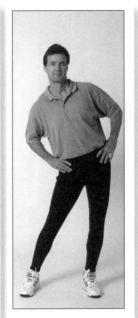 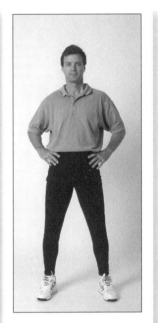

Don't laugh, this is a great way to warm up through the hips. Think it's easy? Well, it was when you were twelve years old. With your hands on your hips, rotate your pelvis in circles. Repeat ten times in each direction.

Muscles used: Hips and waist muscles.

Result: Helps backswing, downswing, and follow through.

Tip: Start with small circles and gradually increase their size.

14. Hamstrings

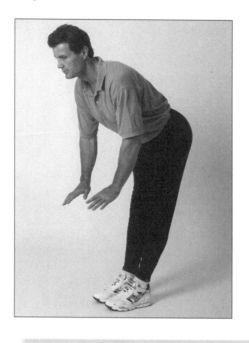

Bend forward at the waist, keeping your stomach tight and your back flat. Do not bounce. Stay where you can feel the stretch and hold for 10 seconds, repeating twice. Tight hamstrings = tight back = tight swing.

Muscles used: Back of leg muscles.

Result: Improves address, backswing, downswing, impact, and follow through and makes walking those 18 holes a little easier.

Tip: It is not how far you go, but how consistent you are with the stretches that will improve your flexibility.

15. Quadriceps

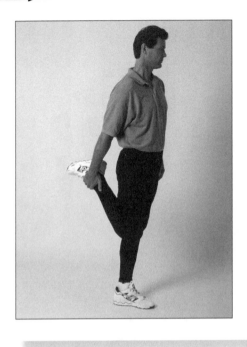

Standing straight, grab your foot or ankle behind you and pull your heel to your butt. Try to keep your knees together. Hold onto a chair or wall if you need additional support. Hold for 10 seconds, and repeat twice with each leg.

Muscles used: Quadricep muscles.

Result: Helps address, backswing, downswing, impact, and follow through.

Tip: By pressing your hips forward, you will increase the stretch in the front of your hips.

---

16. Calves and Achilles Tendons

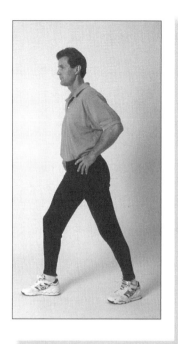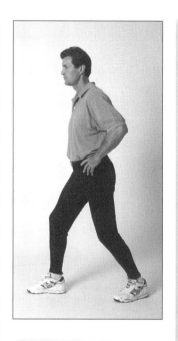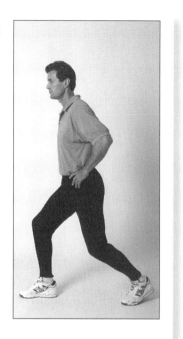

Walking 18 holes can easily fatigue your lower legs. Standing with one foot in front of the other, keep your feet facing forward and press your rear heel on the ground. Feel the stretch in your calves for 10 seconds, repeating twice.

Advanced: Slightly bend your rear knee for an advanced Achilles tendon stretch.

Muscles used: Calf muscles and Achilles tendons.

Result: Improves follow through, prevents Achilles tendonitis, and prepares your calves for impact and walking the course.

Tip: Be careful not to bounce when doing this stretch.

17. Knee and Ankle Rotators

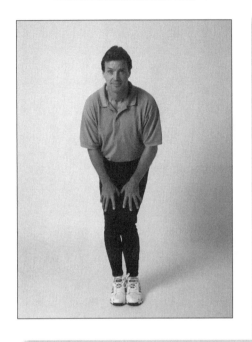 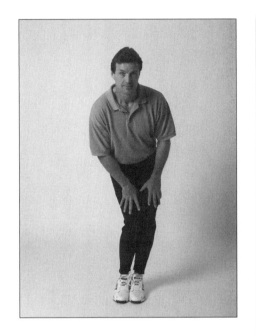

Place your hands on your knees and slightly bend your legs. Keep your knees and feet together as you rotate your knees clockwise and counter-clockwise eight times.

Muscles used: Knee and ankle muscles.

Result: Address, backswing, downswing, impact, and follow through are improved.

Tip: Preparation is crucial for this area. The downswing puts a lot of stress on the knee joints. Start with small circles and work toward larger ones.

18. Inner Thigh

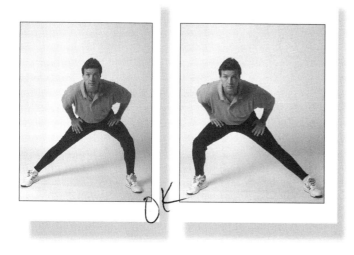

Stand with your feet more than shoulder width apart and rest your hands on your hips or thighs for support. Keep one leg straight while bending the other leg and hold for eight seconds. Switch legs and repeat four times.

Advanced: For a more challenging stretch, place your hands on the floor between your legs.

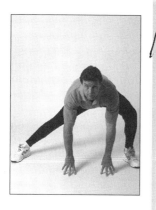
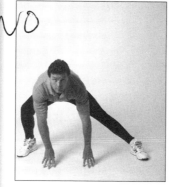

Muscles used: Inner thigh muscles.

Result: Helps backswing and downswing, and prepares the leg muscles for impact with the ball.

Tip: If this stretch is too difficult, try the seated butterfly stretch (see page 44).

19. Hay Balers

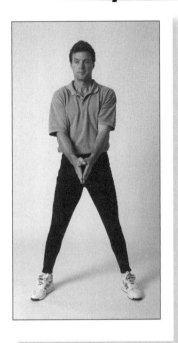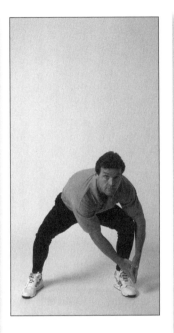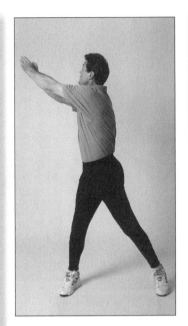

With your feet shoulder width apart and your palms together, stretch your arms straight out in front of you. Drop your hands to your left foot and then up over your right shoulder. Switch sides and repeat ten times.

Muscles used: Lower and upper legs, butt, waist, torso, shoulders, and arms.

Result: Improves address, backswing, downswing, impact, and follow through.

Tip: Hay balers are the final touch to complete our warm-up, combining all the stretches in a synchronized movement. Add one to three pound weights on each hand to increase the intensity of this exercise.

Golf Flex 10-Minute Post-Game Seated Floor Stretches

The following stretches are static and restorative in nature. Hold the stretch position for at least 20 seconds. These are excellent stretches to work on during the week for improving flexibility and health of the hips, shoulders, spine and lower back or to cool down after golf or a workout. They can also help increase joint mobility by applying a gentle rocking motion at the stretch point.

1. Indian Sits
2. Child Pose
3. Butterfly
4. Corkscrews
5. Abdominal and Back Stretch
6. Lower Back Stretch
7. Tinkerbell

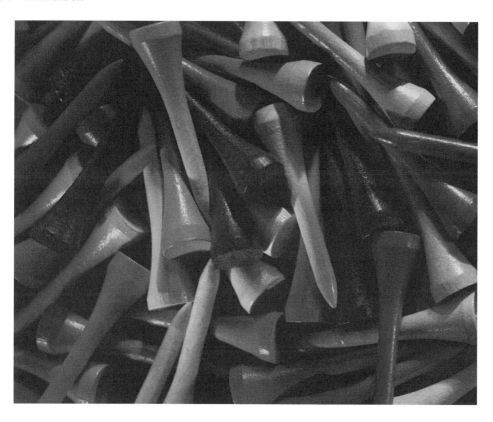

1. Indian Sits

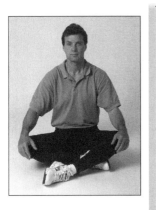
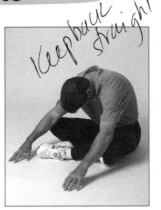

Keep back straight!

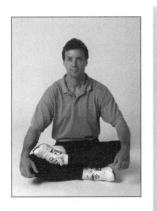
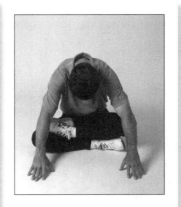

This is a great outer hip stretch. Start by sitting on the floor with your legs crossed, leaving both feet on the ground. Incorporate a back stretch by placing your hands on the floor in front of you. Lower your chin as you walk your hands forward, letting your chest fall to your knees. This is a wonderful multi-purpose exercise, which stretches your hips, butt, shoulders, and back. Alternate sides and repeat.

Advanced: Increase your hip stretch by sitting with one foot over of the opposite knee.

2. Child Pose

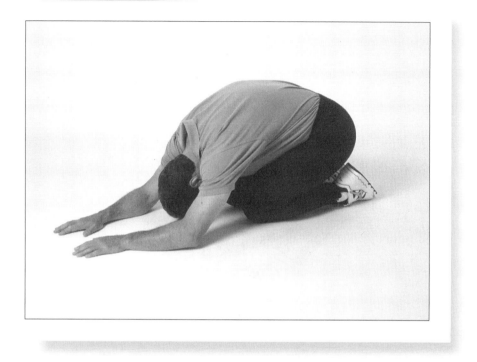

Sit on your heels, drop your chest to your knees, and reach your hands out in front of you. A great relaxing stretch, this exercise stretches your ankles, legs, butt, and back.

3. Butterfly

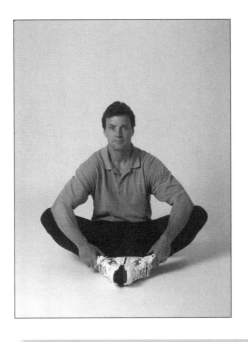

Sit with the soles of your feet together and your knees out to the sides. Hold your ankles as you gently press your knees apart with your elbows. Be careful not to bounce.

4. Corkscrews

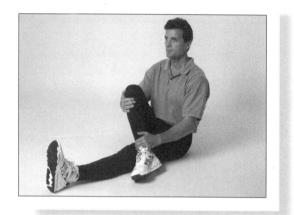

Sit with your left leg straight and cross your right foot over your left leg. It is important to keep your back straight. Do not slouch! Place your right hand behind you, and your left arm outside your right leg. Turn and look toward your right hand. Be sure to pay attention to your breathing. Without changing feet position, turn and face the other direction. Hold each of these positions for 30 seconds. Repeat with the opposite leg.

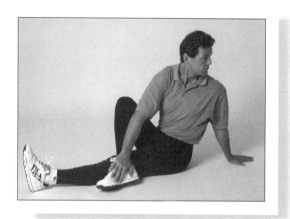

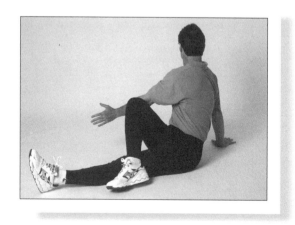

5. Abdominal and Back Stretch

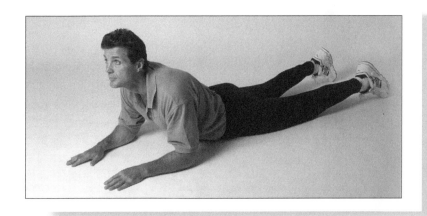

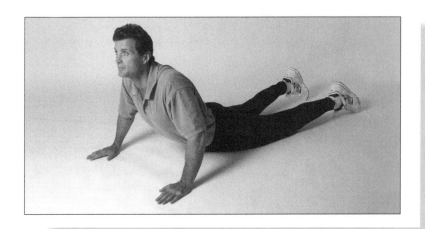

Lie on your stomach and lift your chest up on your elbows. Flex your abdominal muscles as you stretch your back.

Advanced: Lift your entire body up on your hands. This is a much more intense stretch. It is not recommended for those recovering from lower back injuries.

6. Lower Back Stretch

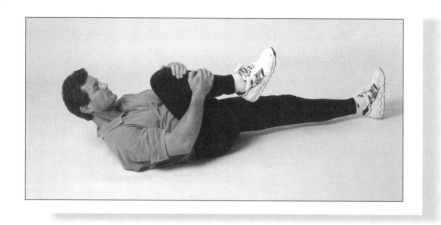

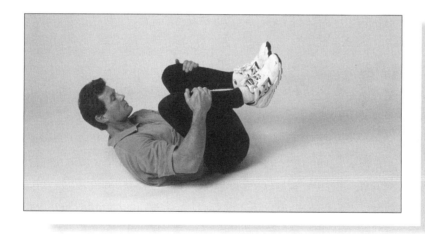

Lie on your back and bend one knee, while keeping the other leg straight. Hold the shin of your bent knee to your chest. Repeat with the opposite leg.

Advanced: For added intensity, hold both shins to your chest.

7. Tinkerbell

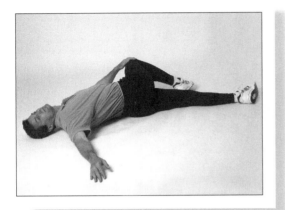

Lying on your back, bend your right knee over the left, keeping your left leg straight. Pull the right leg across with your left hand and look in the opposite direction of the stretch. Reach your right hand out to the side and repeat with the opposite leg.

Advanced: Keep your right leg straight as you cross it over your left leg. Hold both arms out to the sides. Repeat with the opposite leg.

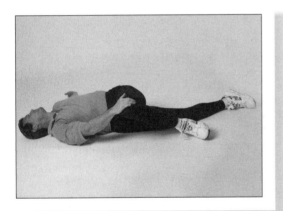

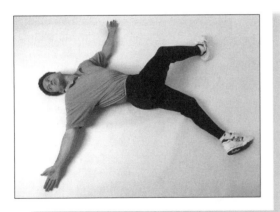

Post-Game Flex

While pre-game stretching warms your muscles, helps avoid injuries, and prepares your body for the movements of golf, post-game stretching alleviates soreness and keeps your muscles from snapping back tighter than they were before the game.

Throughout the Day

"The most important thing is flexibility. Find a good stretching routine and stick to it daily."

—Cameron Doan, PGA Pro

The Golf Flex program is great, but how am I going to stretch during the week? I hardly have time to eat breakfast and kiss the family goodbye. I just don't have time for a flexibility program. This is the beauty of Golf Flex. You can practice your flexibility routine anywhere—at home, in the car, or at the office. Just do a few minutes at a time and you will achieve long-term results.

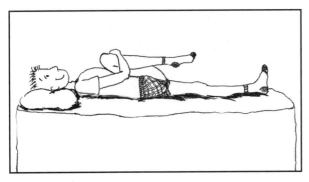

Now let's incorporate these stretches into our daily lives. You will see how easy it is to stretch as you do your everyday tasks, and how quickly your flexibility will increase.

In Bed. Do these stretches before you get out of bed in the morning and your back will love you.

Bring one knee to your chest, hold for 10 seconds, and alternate knees. Then, bring both knees to your chest for 10 seconds. Fold your knees over to one side, then the other side, holding for 10 seconds each. Be sure to keep your shoulders flat on the bed.

As you increase in flexibility, move smoothly from one position to the next. These stretches will warm up, stretch, and prepare your back and spine for the day!

Rise and shine. Give yourself a big hug, stretching your upper and mid back. Hold one arm across your chest and hug it toward you with the opposite hand. Alternate arms, stretching the shoulder muscles.

From either a seated or standing position, interlace your fingers and lift your hands over your head, pushing your palms away from you. This stretches your forearms, shoulders, and ribcage. This exercise can be increased by gently leaning over to one side, stretching your waist. Be sure to keep your abdominal muscles tight while doing this stretch.

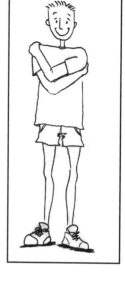

Time to shower. A nice hot shower is an excellent opportunity to warm up and stretch. Start by letting the hot water hit the back of your neck, relaxing your upper back and neck muscles. Slowly do half circles, letting your chin roll from one shoulder to the other. Repeat approximately six times.

Now that your back is warmed up, do a few tree huggers. Let the water run down your upper and mid back. Hold each stretch for 10 seconds. Continue to stretch your back by adding a few back scratchers.

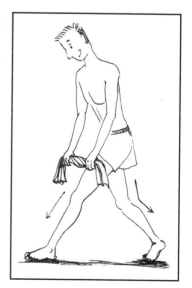

Turn and face the water, letting it warm your chest muscles as you do six rooster crows. You have just gotten a great upper body stretch in no time. Shower everyday, stretch everyday—see the difference it makes!

Toweling off. Grab a towel at both ends, bringing one hand over your head and one behind your back. Reverse the motion and rotate your hands. This is a wonderful way to stretch your rotator cuffs and keep your shoulders healthy.

Stand with one foot forward, bending your rear knee and keeping your front leg straight while you towel off. To increase this stretch, wrap the towel around your forward foot and gently pull towards you. This exercise increases the strength and flexibility of your calves and Achilles tendons.

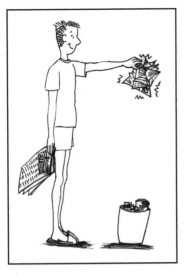

Reading the paper. You do it every morning! Take this time to also strengthen your hands and forearms. After reading a section of the paper, take sheet in one hand and slowly crumble it into a tight ball. This is a lot harder than it seems. Try getting up to four sheets per hand.

Getting dressed. Putting on a T-shirt is something we do everyday and it can be a great stretch for our shoulders, ribcage, and arms. As you put one arm through your shirt, reach as far as you can toward the sky, and repeat with the opposite arm.

Putting on socks and shoes. While seated, cross one ankle over the opposite knee and feel the stretch in the back of your legs and butt as you lean over to put on your sock. Reverse leg position and put on the other sock. Then slip on your shoes. Go down on one knee as you tie your shoe, stretching the front of your hip and your back leg.

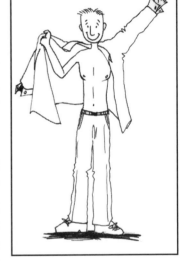

Sitting in the car, waiting for it to warm up. Keep your right hand on the steering wheel and reach your left hand across your body to the back of your seat. This really opens up your back and shoulders. Repeat on the opposite side.

Interlace both hands behind your head and reach backward, stretching both your chest and back.

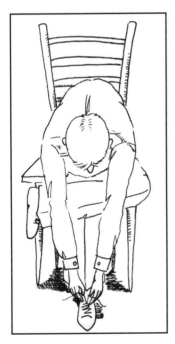

At the office. For many, sitting at the office all day can make us tight and often tense. Sitting with our legs crossed for hours at a time while hunched over our desks, does nothing to promote flexibility. However, taking just a few minutes a day, you can easily increase your well-being and flexibility. There is an old Italian saying, "Chi va piano va sano e lontano," meaning, "He who goes slow, goes safely and far." A little every day will get you results!

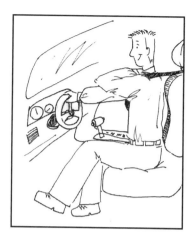

Sit with your left ankle over your right knee. Keeping your spine straight, place your right hand on your left knee, and turn your torso to your left. In the same seated position, turn your torso to the right by placing your left hand on the outside of your right thigh. This is a great spine stretch! Continue by placing both hands on your thighs and gently lower your chest toward your knees, stretching your butt, back, and thighs. Reverse feet position and repeat.

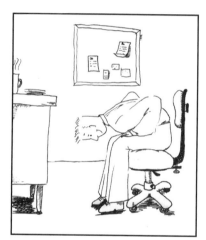

Sit with your feet flat on the floor and slowly drop your head between your knees, letting your hands fall to the floor. You will feel this stretch in your lower back and butt. While in this stretch position, remember to breathe deeply into your lower back, filling your lungs and slowly letting tension release with each exhale.

Grab both sides of the doorway with your hands at shoulder level. Walk forward until you feel the stretch in your arms. This exercise is great for your chest and shoulder muscles.

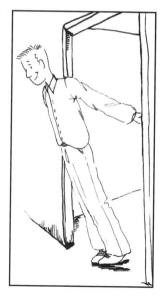

The following stretches can also be done seated at your desk:

- Yes and No
- Peach Pickers
- Willow Tree

Part V:
Golf Flex Injury
Hot Spots and Prevention

WHILE MUSCLE OVERUSE IS A COMMON CAUSE OF INJURY for professional golfers, weekend golfers' injuries are most often a result of improper form, muscle weakness, and lack of flexibility.

You will notice the back, abs, and hips are included in the following injury prevention exercises. These areas are sometimes referred to as the power zone. In any sport that requires the motion of throwing or swinging, this part of the body stabilizes and generates power from your trunk to your torso.

Injury Hot Spots

Elbows/Wrist/Forearms—Gripping the club often results in impact and overuse injuries.

Shoulders—The shoulders are the most common area injured in any sport that involves throwing or swinging.

Back—The golf swing can cause major strain from the neck to the lower back.

Hips—If your hips are tight, you will not generate rotation power; and if your back is tight, your hips will overcompensate, causing overuse injuries.

Feet/Ankles—Walking 18 holes can cause soreness in the front of your ankle and the soles of your feet, and also may result in shin splints.

Golfer's Elbow

In the medical profession this is known as medial epicondylitis, and yes, it does mean pain. Golfer's elbow is a form of tendonitis. Tendons are the ends of muscles that attach to the bone. This particular tendon is the bony point where the muscles of the forearm that flex the wrist originate. Inflammation can cause pain all down the forearm when gripping an object. This form of tendonitis is most commonly caused by overused tendons and/or improper technique.

The recommended treatment is **R.I.C.E.**: Rest, Ice, Compression and Elevation.

Rest—to prevent further injury and relieve stress from the area of discomfort.

Ice—reduce swelling by decreasing circulation to the area.

Compression—bracing or wrapping the injured area to reduce expanding and swelling.

Elevation—to decrease the amount of blood and fluid to the irritated area.

Depending on its severity, golfer's elbow can take six weeks or longer to heal. It is important to see a doctor for a proper diagnosis. Once the inflammation is reduced, you can incorporate stretching and strengthening exercises. The biggest mistake most people make is not resting long enough. Coming back too soon can result in re-injury and further damage. The key to recovery is rest.

Taking an anti-inflammatory can be helpful if you have no ulcers or contraindication to this medication.

Fortunately, as a recreational golfer you can afford to rest. Many that suffer from medial epicondylitis are workmen that refuse to take time off. Refusing to rest can cause scarring and permanent damage. Although rare, surgeries are performed in about 10-15% of severe cases.

Lay down the golf club at the first sign of pain. Begin a regime of icing and stretching the forearm. A simple method to ice is to keep a small paper cup filled with water in the freezer. Gently massage and ice your elbow twice day. Stretch and flex your forearm by gently pressing your hand into flexion and extension.

Once the pain goes away, and this can take up to several months in severe cases, begin a strengthening program for your forearms. Have a golf pro review your swing to insure your technique is not at fault. Stretch your forearms as part of your pre-game warm-up. Finally be sure to strengthen your core, as a strong core is the power base for rotation. A strong core will reduce the stress, which can be absorbed in the arms.

Back Pain

It's a lucky golfer or anyone over 18 that at one time or another has not experienced back pain. Approximately 70 to 90 percent of our population suffers with low back pain. Back pain is a complex problem that can be brought on by several factors such as age, lifestyle, diet, dehydration, stress, daily living activity, or a sports related injury.

You can help avoid and or control back pain by keeping yourself physically fit, hydrated, maintaining your flexibility, cardio conditioning, and core strength training. A body out of balance has a higher risk of injury.

Golfers can also develop back problems when they stop golfing or exercising consistently. Becoming de-conditioned will increase your risk of back injury. During the off season is the perfect time to maintain a fitness program, so when you do golf it doesn't feel it's "too much too fast."

Even active golfers injure their backs with repetitive movements that cause over-use injuries. Though many golfers might squirm at the idea of exercise that doesn't consist of being on the green, they would be even more miserable if they couldn't bend over to pick up a ball.

If you suffer from back pain, go to a health practitioner who can design a functional exercise program that takes into consideration your entire body. Back injuries are complex and they need to be properly diagnosed or you could do yourself more harm than good.

According to the American Academy of Orthopedic Surgeons, anywhere from 45% to 80% of golfers experience lower back pain. In 1991, there were 7,000 reported golf injuries; by 1998 this figure had doubled to 14,000. To avoid musculoskeletal injuries, the AAOS recommended warm-up and flexibility training before playing.

Here are three common types of back injuries:

Lumbar disc derangement is commonly known as a "slipped disc." This occurs when the center (nucleus) of the disc begins to bulge out against the surrounding (annulus fibrosis). The level of pain and discomfort depends on which of four stages of disc derangement one has. Movements involving forward flexion like picking up a ball without proper abdominal support, poor posture, and the constant rotation required by golfing can often cause it. It is normally seen in people ages 20 to 50. Back extension exercises help this condition, as well as strong core exercises that stabilize the paraspinal muscles of the back. Your health practitioner should design these for you.

Ankylosing spondylitis is a defect in the area between the vertebra facets called pars interasticularis. It can be genetic or caused by forceful hyperextension. It is typically seen in individuals between 20 and 30 but can also occur in young athletes active in explosive sports like gymnastics, tennis, diving, football, ice hockey, and golf. Back extension exercises would be very painful and not to be performed under this condition.

Spinal stenosis is the narrowing of the spinal canal, which contains and protects the spinal cord and nerve roots. This results in low back pain and perhaps leg pain. Stenosis can be acquired from wear and tear, faulty loading, or even can be congenital. It is often seen in individuals over 50 years old with past back injuries. Forward flexion exercises are good for this condition.

Beyond Stretching: Myofascial Release

Have you ever felt a knot between your shoulder blades or upper back that no amount of stretching will release? Do your legs feel as tight as a piano strings or are your calves chronically sore after walking 18 holes? Then you might find relief with a self-message technique done with a foam roller (cost less than $20 at www.performbetter.com) and your own body weight.

The body's muscles, nerves and blood vessels are encased in a tissue called fascia. Fascia is found throughout the body and, when it is restricted because of injury, inflexibility, or overuse, the muscles will bind and cause pain. This will reduce your range of motion, increase tightness, create soft tissue adhesions and muscle soreness. This then results in an injury cycle of movement compensations, poor movement patterns, and early muscle fatigue which can destroy the consistency of your golf swing.

By using a foam roller before or after a golf round you can alleviate or release these fascial restrictions.

How You Do It

1. Maintain each position and roll along the roller for 1 to 2 minutes at a time.
2. When you reach a painful spot, stop the roller and hold the position for 30 to 40 seconds.
3. Be sure to keep your abs braced, keeping good posture and maintain an even breath flow.

These self-release techniques can be done once or twice a day.

Hot Spots

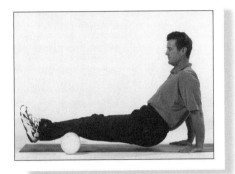

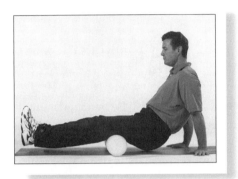

Calves. Place the back of your calves on the roller. Lift your hips off of the floor and roll both sides of your calves. Keep your feet relaxed. For a more intense massage, cross one leg over the other and apply pressure with the top leg.

Hamstrings. Place the back of your thighs on the roller. Roll from your knees to your hips. Tightening the quadriceps while rolling on the hamstrings will increase the massage.

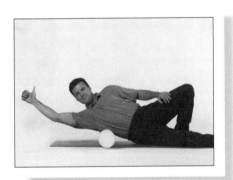

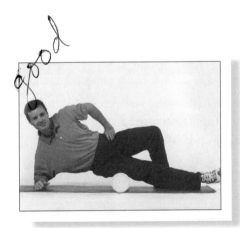

Latissimus Dorsi. Place the side of your chest on the roller. With your arm extended over your head, point your thumb up.

IT Band. Place the outside of your bottom thigh on the roller. Bend top leg and place it on the floor for stabilization. Roll from your hips to your knee.

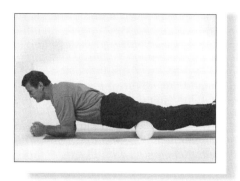

Quadriceps. Place the fronts of your thighs on the roller. Roll from your hips to your knees.

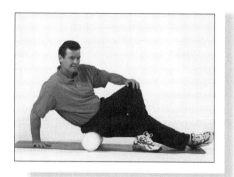

Piriformis. Sit on the roller with one foot crossed over the opposite knee.

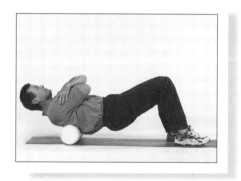

Rhomboids. Place your shoulder blades on roller. Fold your arm across your chest and lift your hips off of the floor for increased pressure.

Forearm and Hand Strengthening

"We need our wrists and forearms to be flexible."

—John Buczek, PGA Pro

Try some of these simple and effective stretching and strengthening exercises to help prevent golfer's elbow.

Hand Squeeze—Spread open your hand, then make a tight fist. Continue to open and close your hands, working up to 50 times.

Hand Squeeze With Resistance—Using a pliable rubber ball or old tennis ball, squeeze and release your fist. Keep a ball handy at your desk and do this exercise throughout the day.

Sand Gripping—Fill a bucket with sand and shove your hand in up to your wrist. Keep your hand in the sand as you open and close your fist. This is one tough exercise, but it will give you great results!

Let's begin where the tires hit the road—the hands, wrists, and forearms. Any weakness here will surely result in golfer's elbow. Strengthening the hands will give you the control needed to improve your game and avoid injury.

As mentioned earlier, a simple way to incorporate hand strengthening exercises into your day can be done while reading the newspaper. Taking one sheet at a time, use one hand to crumple the page into a tight ball. Do three or four sheets a day and you will notice an increased hand grip. When you swing, your wrists and hands work to generate power and control the golf club.

Strengthening the Rotator Cuffs

One of the most complex joints in the body, most of us are not even sure what rotator cuffs are. The rotators, commonly called rotator cuffs, are four little muscles that stabilize your arms and shoulders during your golf swing. Many golfers suffer from shoulder injuries due to weak or strained rotator cuffs. If you want to stay in the game, it is crucial to maintain healthy rotators. Here are four simple stretching and strengthening exercises to keep your rotator cuffs and shoulders happy and healthy.

Tips

1. Always stretch after performing these exercises.
2. Use a pillow or rolled up towel to support your head if you feel neck strain.
3. Work in slow and controlled movements.
4. Use a full range of motion.

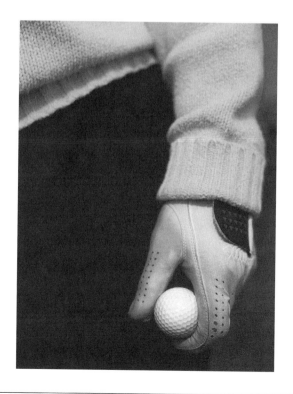

1. Bye-Byes

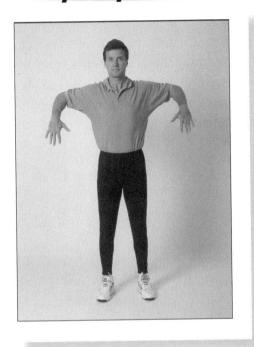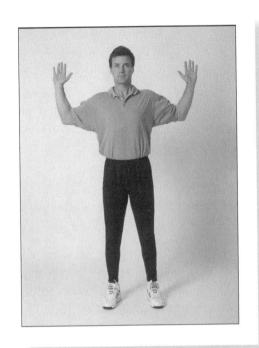

With your arms out to the sides, bend your forearms up from the elbows 90 degrees with your palms facing forward. Then, rotate your forearms, pressing your palms down. Repeat eight times. Keep your shoulders stable and only rotate your arms. Work smoothly and slowly.

2. External Rotations

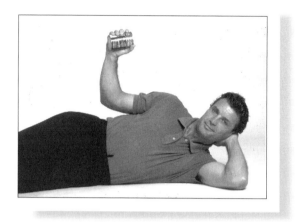

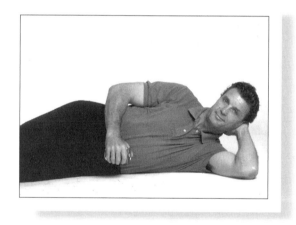

Lie on your side with your legs together and your knees bent. Place your bottom arm behind your head for support and your top arm at your waist, bent 90 degrees. Rotate your forearm from your stomach straight up and repeat on the other side. Start with three sets of 20, using one- to three-pound weights and work up to five pounds.

3. Internal Rotations

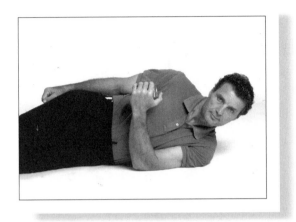

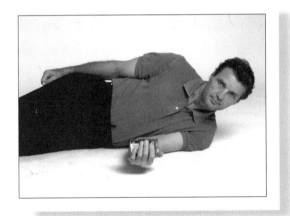

Lie on your side with your legs together and your knees bent. Rest on your shoulder with your top arm at your hip, and your bottom arm bent 90 degrees. Rotate your bottom arm from your stomach to the floor and repeat on the other side. Start with three sets of 20 using one- to three-pound weights and work up to five pounds.

Lower Back

"Eight percent of all golfers will incur some sort of back pain during their golf careers."

—Dr. Jim Suttie, PGA M.D.

The back takes on such a tremendous amount of stress during the golf swing that it is no wonder the lower back is a major source of injury for golfers. Before engaging in a back strengthening and stretching program, it is important to consult your doctor. The back is a complex area. Problems can arise from stress, poor posture, and certainly poor mechanics of the golf swing.

To maintain and condition your lower back, it is essential to keep it strong and flexible. The following are back strengthening exercises. They should be done in conjunction with abdominal exercises. Strengthening your abdominal muscles is an essential part of maintaining an overall healthy and strong back. The abdominal muscles help stabilize the back, while the obliques rotate your torso during your swing. No back conditioning program is complete without abdominal exercises.

Back Exercises

1. Superman

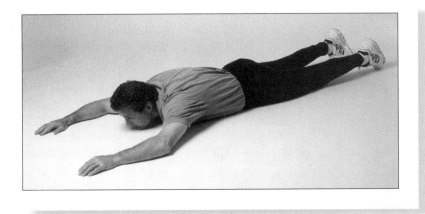

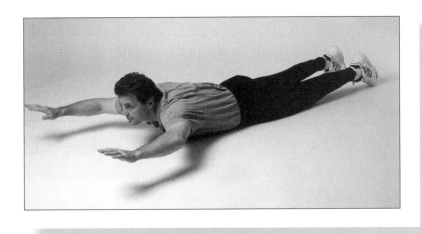

Lie on your stomach and extend your arms in front of you. Lift your chest and arms off the ground.

GOLF FLEX

2. Lois Lane

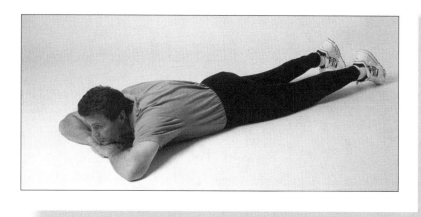

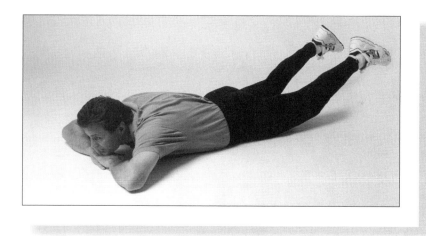

Lie on your stomach with your hands under your chin. Keep your chest on the floor as you lift your thighs and feet.

Back Exercises

3. Swimmer

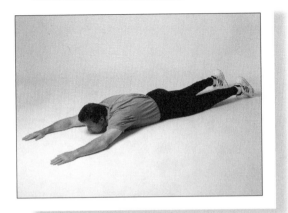

In the same position as the superman stretch, lift your right arm and left leg. Repeat with the opposite arm and leg.

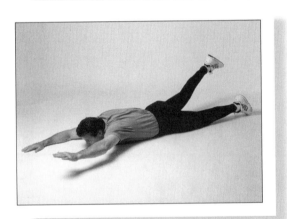

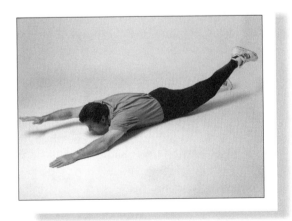

Glute and Lower Back Stretch

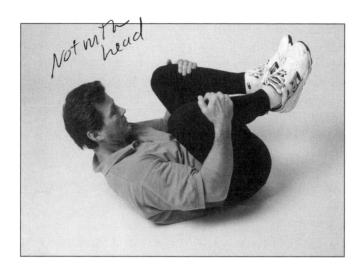

TIP
Holding your knees to your chest is a great way to give your back an overall stretch after exercising.

Seated stretches that add flexibility to your back:

1. Indian Sits
2. Child Pose
3. Butterfly
4. Corkscrews
5. Abdominal and Back Stretch
6. Lower Back Stretch
7. Tinkerbell

Abdominal Exercises

1. Standard Crunch

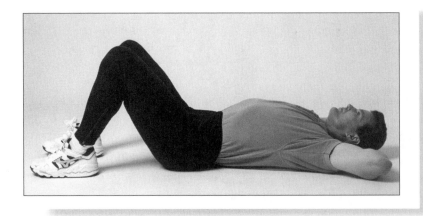

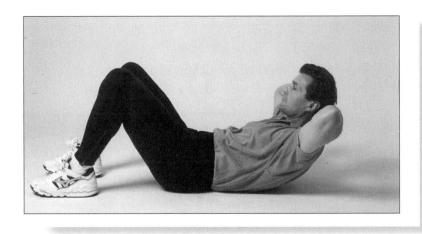

Lie on your back with your knees bent. With your hands behind your head, contract your abdominal muscles and lift your shoulders off the floor. Be careful not to pull on your neck.

2. Oblique Crunches

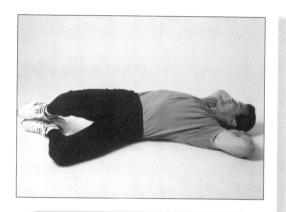

Lie on your back with your knees together to one side, and lift your shoulders off the floor. Repeat on both sides.

TIP
Keeping your elbows flat, not pointed, reduces the strain on your neck.

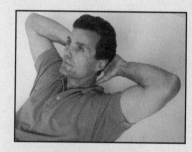

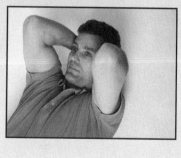

Abdominal Exercises

3. Reverse Curls

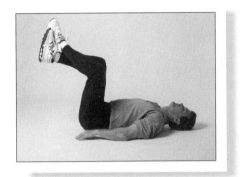

Lie on your back with your knees and feet in the air, and place your hands on the floor at your sides. Lift your hips off the ground and tilt your pelvis up toward your chest. Do not bounce or jerk. Cross your feet for additional comfort.

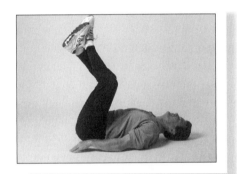

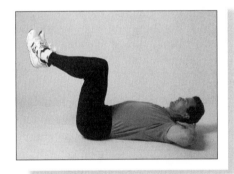

Advanced: With your hands behind your head, lift your hips, shoulders, and head.

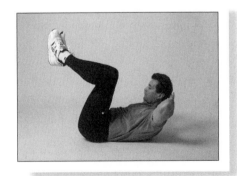

Hips

"Good hip rotation promises a good swing."

Linda Mulherin, PGA Pro

The most important part of the power zone, strong and flexible hips will keep you in the game and prevent nagging strains. Fortunately, we have many opportunities throughout the day to stretch our hips. Putting on your socks is a great way to work the sides of your hips, lacing your shoes works the front, and bending over while seated at your desk works the inner thighs.

Here are a few simple thigh and hip strengthening exercises.

Hip Exercises

1. Scissors

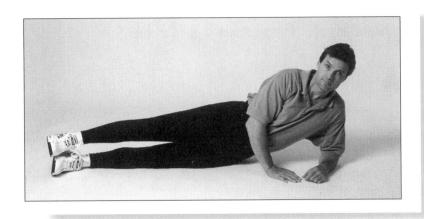

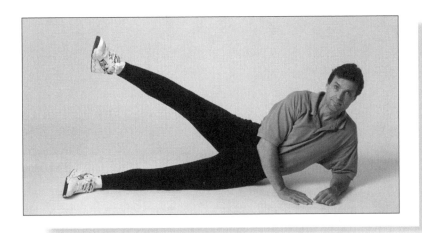

Lie on your side with your legs straight, and lift your top leg away from your bottom leg. Repeat on both sides.

2. Inner Thigh

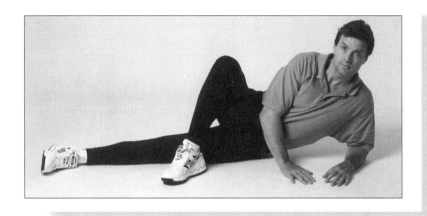

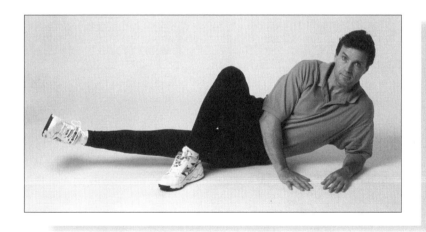

On your side, cross one foot over the other leg and lift the straight leg six inches off the ground. Repeat on both sthides.

Hip Exercises

3. Standing Squats

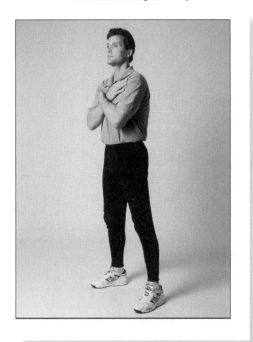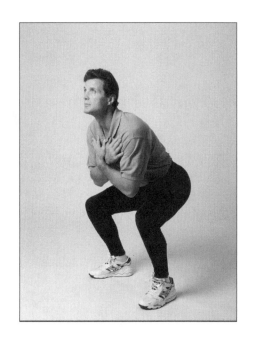

Stand with your feet shoulder width apart. Cross your arms against your chest and keep your heels solid on the ground. Drop your butt back as though you were sitting in a chair. Keep your chest high and shoulders back as you try to keep your butt level with your knees.

Feet and Ankles

You can't play golf if you're not on your feet. The feet are your base of balance and power. Try throwing a baseball sitting in a chair.

A quick calves and Achilles stretch helps to prepare your calf muscles and Achilles tendons for walking 18 holes. Stretch the front of your ankles by sitting on the heel of your foot on the floor. Do the same stretch standing as you gently roll your foot forward. You can even do this stretch while on the course. A great way to massage aching feet and prevent plantar fasciitis, or heel spurs, is to stretch after a game. Your feet will love you for it!

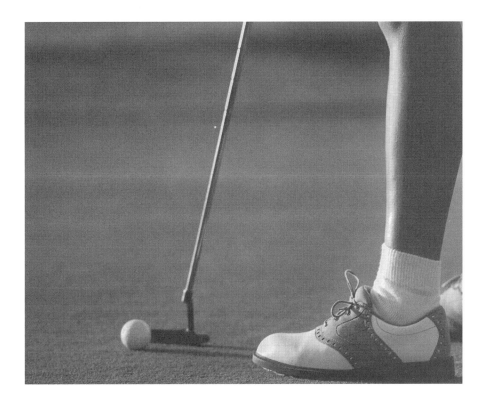

Part VI:
Golf Flex Strength Program: 30 Minutes To A More Powerful Game

TRAINING ON A EXERCISE BALL HAS MANY UNIQUE BENEFITS. Conventional weight training on machines at the gym strengthens your big muscles or primary movers, but neglect the, smaller postural muscles. The exercise ball is ideal for strength training because it forces you to engage your core and stabilizing muscles. It also trains your muscles to move in integration not isolation. At the same time, training on an exercise ball will increase awareness of your balance and equilibrium. As we grow older, our balance systems become less sensitive. In addition, free weights such as dumbbells allow you to exercise in movement pathways that are specific to your body type, and not ones forced by a machine.

Strength training should not be confused with bodybuilding. You will not be ripping through your shirt like the Hulk. You will get stronger and leaner and develop a platform in which to create more power and endurance because you will be developing real strength. Real or functional strength is the strength you can manage without external support (bench or machine). Since the ball is an unstable surface, it will force you to use your own body as a stabilizer, so the strength you create is strength you can use.

With strength training you will also reduce your body fat and increase your metabolism. As we age, our muscles naturally atrophy and our bone density decreases. We can prevent both of these with strength training. A solid 30-minute strength program can increase your metabolism for 14 to 48 hours, unlike cardio training that ceases to burn calories the moment you stop exercising. You've heard the old adage "use it or lose it." It's true. For example, if you broke your arm the doctor would put it in a cast. The cast when first applied is tight, but within weeks it becomes loose. Either (A)the cast stretches or (B)your muscles atrophy, and it's not A.

Core Strength

The core is your abdominals and your lower back. Like cables to a bridge, the core must be strong to maintain the integrity and stability of the trunk. A strong core is the link that connects movements between your hips and your shoulders during your golf swing.

Your core is the center of power. It's also where your center of gravity is. It plays an essential role in your balance and equilibrium. It is involved in respiration and provides intra-abdominal pressure, thus protecting your spine and lower back. A strong and healthy core is optimal for good posture. It is essential in the reduction of overuse and wear and tear of your joints. A strong and stable core will make you feel, perform and look better. What good would it do to have strong legs, shoulders, arms and chest, if you can strain your back when you bend over to pick up a ball?

To properly train your core we will need a basic understanding of anatomy and how the abdominal and lower back muscles function. The abdominal unit is made up of four muscles, the *rectus abdominis, external oblique, internal oblique,* and the *transverse.* The rectus abdominis (commonly known as your six pack) originates at the pubic bone crest and is inserted in the ribs next to the solarplex. The rectus stabilizes your spine and assists in forward flexion. The external oblique is the largest of the abdominal muscles. It is located at the fifth to the twelfth ribs, running straight down the linea alba. It rotates the trunk from side to side, anchored by the opposing internal oblique. The internal oblique lies inferior to the external oblique. It originates at the middle of the top of the hip bone (iliac crest) and is inserted in the tenth, eleventh, and twelfth ribs. It's responsible for same-side flexion. It is important that the external and the opposing internal oblique work together to create a powerful rotation of the trunk.

Seated deeply beneath all these muscles is the very important transverse abdominis. It originates in the lower back and is inserted in the center of the rectus. The TVA is the only abdominal muscle with muscle fibers that are horizontal. It is the major stabilizer of the lumbar spine, and it acts as the body's natural weight belt. Often ignored, it is essential to have a TVA that can protect and maintain a healthy back.

Strengthening Your TVA

The large back muscles along the spine are known as the *erector spinae muscle group* (spinalis, longisimus, and illocostalis) counterbalance the forward flexion of the abdominal musculature. These muscles run up the vertebral column and are responsible for extension and side flexion of the spine. While performing back extensions on the exercise ball you will also encourage an important myriad of smaller, deeper synergistic muscles (multifidus) along the spine to activate and increase stabilization among the vertebrae. This is an extremely important and often neglected portion of strengthening the core. A core strengthening program is not complete without including strengthening these back muscles, in fact you would be encouraging poor posture if you did so.

The exerciseball is ideal for abdominal training because its unstable and round surface allows for a greater degree of extension. This added movement trains the muscles through their fullest range of motion, which recruits more muscle fiber. The more muscles recruited the more horsepower you can put into your swing. The unstable nature of the ball requires you to stay alert and maintain a sense of equilibrium.

Flexibility is an important part of any workout, and training your core is no exception. A thorough stretch of the abs and back after a workout will ensure that no muscles become too tight. Tight abdominals can pull down on the front of the ribs and create a forward shoulder posture that might even affect your breathing.

Test Your TVA

Stand with your feet shoulder width apart. Place a coin on the floor a few inches in front of your feet. Place an index finger at your belly button. Bend over and pick up the coin with your opposite hand. What did your belly button do? Did it feel as if it was moving outward, inward, or staying the same? If it was not moving inward, try the following exercise to strengthen and awaken your TVA. ·

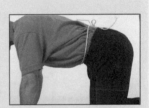

Get on your knees, and reach down to place your hands on the floor. Your hands should be directly under your shoulders and your knees should be directly under your hips. Be sure your waist is bare. Place a light rope or thread around your waist so that it lightly touches the skin of your belly as you inhale. Draw your belly away from the rope during your exhalation so that it is loose. Hold for ten seconds, and repeat 5 to 8 times. Make sure your back and shoulders do not move.

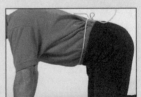

Exercises For Stretching and Strengthening

We have by nature some muscles which are prone to becoming tight and others that are prone to becoming weak. The following is a list of the most common. We cannot allow gravity, age, or repetitive movements to negatively influence our posture.

Tightness

Muscles commonly in need of stretching:

- Flexor of elbow: Bicep Stretch
- Chest (pectoralis major): Chest Stretch
- Outer Hip(tensor faciate latae): MyoFascial Release on Foam Roller
- Upper Back: Upper Back Stretch
- Lats: MyoFascial Release on Foam Roller/Shoulder Stretch
- Hamstrings and Calves: Hamstring and Calf Stretch/MyoFascial Release on Foam Roller

Weakness

Muscles commonly in need of strengthening:

- Serratus Anterior: Chest Press
- Rectus: Core Sets
- Inner Thigh (vastus): The Lift
- Buttock (glute max and medial):Russian Twist or the Outer Thigh Lift
- Extensor of elbow: Tabletop Triceps Extension

Posture Is Power

If you have poor posture, and you begin your strength training program, you will increase your physical deficits. Poor posture increases potential overuse injuries, accelerates wear and tear on our joints, reduces playing performance, and sets you on a fast track to arthritis. A 140 pound man's head weighs about 11 pounds. If he has a forward head posture of about 3 1/2 inches, his head would feel more like 15 1/2 pounds. If he slouched from forward from the waist and trunk by 7.6 degrees, the combined weight of the head and torso would seem like 138 pounds! Think how exhausting or even impossible would be carrying all that extra weight around and how much stress it would put on the spine. Forty years ago when women of villages in Italy would do their laundry on a washing stone then place it all in a basket and carry this load (20-30 pounds) on their head. Do you think they'd be able to do so if they had forward head posture? But now, thanks to our modern way of life, our posture has deteriorated. Sitting down all day does not encourage good posture.

The common characteristics of poor posture:

• bending at the waist rather than the hips
• rounding or hunching over the shoulders to get the arms out in front of the body
• drooping the head and tucking the chin to look down at the ball

You might not have given posture much thought but it is where our movements begin and end. It can affect our ability to breathe properly, play sports, and it definitely affects how we look and feel about ourselves. Improving one's posture first begins with awareness.

To improve your posture I recommend we should look into a 2-part strategy. First we do a low-tech assessment your posture. Then with the knowledge you've gained, choose which are the proper exercises or stretches to use, and which are the ones to avoid.

Before moving on to the assessment, let's take a look at the spine and the anatomy of proper posture. You spine is shaped like an S. It has a forward curve in the lower spine (lumbar), a backward curve in the upper-mid back (thoracic), and another forward curve at the neck (cervical). For optimal rotation, these curves should not be over curved or too flat. If they are abnormal, it will limit range of motion and lock your body.

Low Tech Assessment: Slump or Sway? Stand about a few inches from a wall. Your buttock (tailbone), back of your shoulders (thoracic spine), and back of your head should be in contact with the wall. If you have a normal spine you will have a space behind your lower back (lumbar spine) and the back of your neck (cervical spine). Slide one hand through the curvature in your lower back. The palm of your hand should fit snugly through the curve. If your hand doesn't fit, there's a good chance you're a swayer. If you have too much space or curvature in your lower back, you may have excessive lordosis spine. This can create pressure and strain in the lower back and lumbar disk.

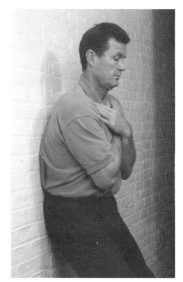

SLUMP

The back of your head should touch the wall without it having to tilt backwards. If you must tilt your head backwards, you probably have excessive curvature of the thoracic spine, known as kyphosis. This commonly creates forward head and shoulder posture. This can result in strain of the disk and muscles of the neck. It can also create shoulder impingement.

Note: Should you discover your posture is out of the norm according to the low tech assessment, you should seek advice from your health practitioner.

Forward Head Posture

1. When standing, practice tucking your chin to your chest.
2. Strengthen your neck by doing Yes and Nos with slight hand resistance.
3. Focus on keeping your chest high and your shoulders back.

Kyphotic Spine

1. Roll a towel so that it is approximately 6 inches around. Lay on the floor and place it behind your shoulders. Lift your arms overhead. Hold for 30 to 60 seconds 4 to 6 times.
2. Stretch your chest and shoulders and strengthen your back.

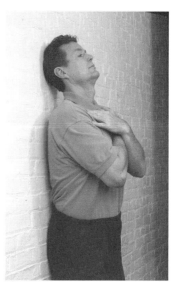

SWAY

Sway back

1. Stretch your hamstrings.
2. Avoid hamstring strengthening exercises.
3. Do Pelvic Tilts on the Exercise Ball.
4. Visually imagine your hips tilting forward and your chest raised high.

Forward Shoulder Posture

1. Stretch your chest.
2. Stretch your abs.
3. Avoid chest strengthening exercises.
4. Strengthen the upper back and rear shoulders.
5. Visually imagine placing your shoulder blades down and in a seated position and your chest raised high.

Warm-Ups

Your exercise ball workout should always begin with a good warm-up. It's never a good idea to start a routine without first slowly raising the body's temperature and thus muscle-tendon suppleness, which enhances balance, ability to shift weight, and improves coordinated movements. This will also help prevent injuries. In addition to the following, you may include any cool-down exercises. Simply perform them in a dynamic fashion.

Standing Rotations

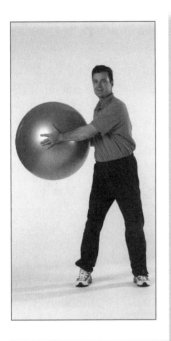 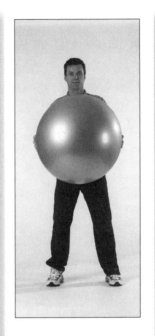 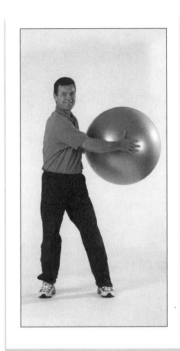

Stand with your feet shoulder width apart and your knees slightly bent. Keep your belly pulled in tightly and your shoulders in their seated position. Hold the ball in your hands with your arms extended. Slowly rotate the ball in a horizontal line from right to left. Don't turn your head; keep your eyes forward.

Draw your belly button toward your spine and keep your abdominals tight throughout this exercise.

Supine Twist

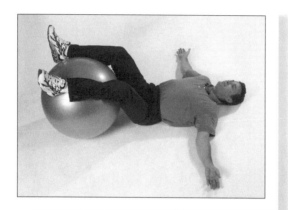

Lay face up on the floor with your arms out to the sides. Place your calves on the ball. Slowly rotate the ball in a small arc from left to right. Keep your shoulders on the floor. As you increase the range of rotation, gently rotate your head in the opposite direction of your knees.

Do not force an increase of your range of motion. Allow your breath and gravity to naturally increase the range of motion.

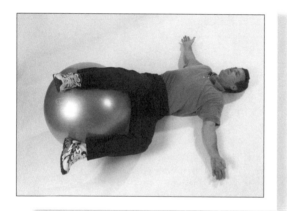

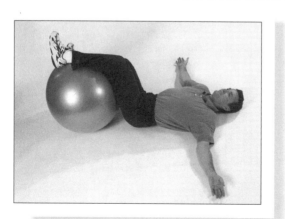

Pelvic Tilts

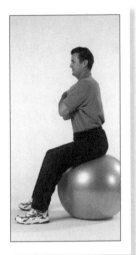 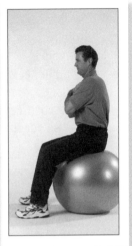 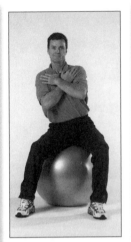 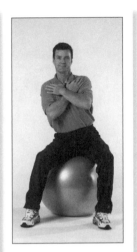

Sit on the apex of the ball with your feet shoulder width apart. Put your hands out to your sides or folded across your chest. Gently rock your pelvis forward and backward. (You might find you have a limited range of movement. That's okay; moving as little as 1 inch is beneficial.) Your ears, shoulders, and hips should be directly in line.

Then, let your hands and arms hang by your side. Make small circles with your hips. Do several in each direction.

Cool-Downs

After you are finished exercising, it's a wise idea to do some cool-down routines. Cooling down after exercise helps avoid fainting or dizziness, which can occur when the exercise is vigorous and is stopped suddenly. A cool-down routine will also help to remove waste products such as lactic acid from your muscles. Slow static stretching is best when the muscles are warm. It will relax your muscles, restore them to their resting length, and gradually improve your range of motion.

Chest Stretch

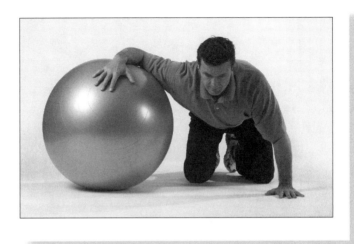

Kneel on the floor with the ball on your right side. Place your right hand and forearm on the ball with your elbow bent at 90-degrees. Roll the ball backward and move your body forward so that your chest goes toward the floor. Hold 2 to 3 seconds and repeat on both sides.

Try extending your arm and moving the ball in various positions to target different muscle fibers.

Shoulder Stretch

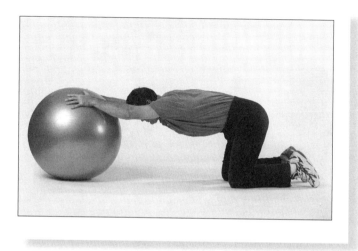

Kneel in front of the ball and place both hands on top of it. Roll the ball forward (your chest will move toward the floor). Then roll the ball to the left and the right to stretch different muscle fibers.

Pay attention to your breathing as you perform this stretch. People often hold their breath as they stretch. Proceed with caution if you have ever had a shoulder injury.

Biceps Stretch

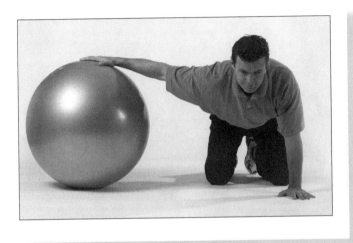

Kneel on the floor with the ball on your right side. Place your right hand on top of the ball. Roll the ball backward and move your body forward so that your chest draws toward the floor.

Hold 2 to 3 seconds and repeat on both sides.

You can avoid stress on your wrists while doing this stretch by keeping your fingers spread wide and distributing your weight throughout your hands and fingers.

Triceps Stretch

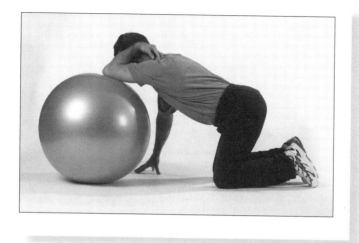

Kneel in front of the ball. Place the back of your upper arm on the ball and press it gently forward until you feel a stretch in your triceps.

For protection, place a rolled-up towel or a pad under your knees whenever you are in a kneeling position.

Waist Stretch

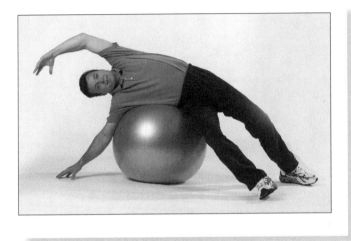

Sit on the apex of the ball, and then walk your feet forward until you're lying on the top of the ball. This position stretches the internal and external obliques—the long sheet of muscle that runs down the middle of your abdomen. Hold for 2 or 3 seconds. From this position, rotate to one side and reach the top arm over your head. Keep your feet wide apart for balance. Hold 2 to 3 seconds. This segment of the position stretches your waist.

Changing the leg position will alter the stretch from the front to the back of the waist.

Back Stretch

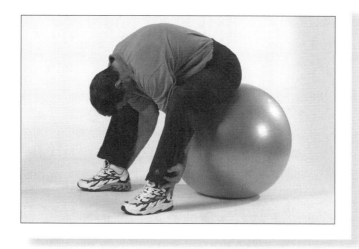

Sit on the apex of the ball with your feet wide apart and flat on the floor. Lower your head between your knees and reach your hands toward the floor. Keep your neck and shoulders relaxed. Hold 2 to 3 seconds and repeat.

For a deeper stretch, wrap your arms around the inside of your calves.

Upper Back Stretch

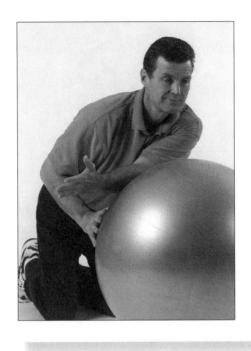

Kneel in front of the ball. Place the arm that is across your chest onto the ball and gently apply downward pressure on the arm. You will feel the stretch behind the upper back and shoulder.

Changing the angle to which you apply pressure will target different muscle fibers of the back.

Quadriceps Stretch

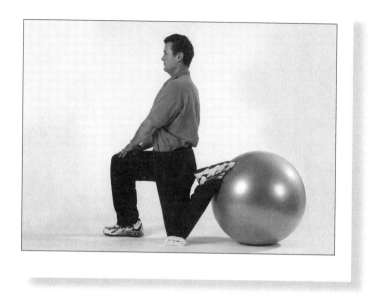

Place one knee on the floor, then place the instep of that foot on the ball. Hold 2 to 3 seconds and repeat. You'll feel the stretch in the front of your thigh.

To increase this stretch and stretch the hips flexor, press your hips away from the ball. If you're less flexible, try a smaller ball; if you're more flexible, a larger.

Hamstrings and Calf Stretch

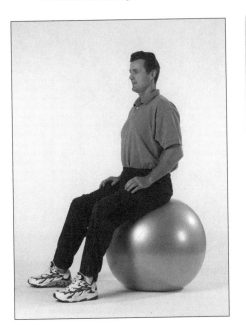 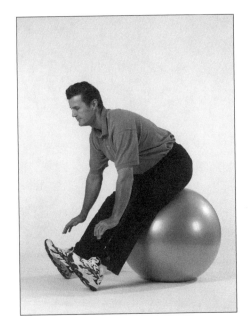

Sit on the apex of the ball with your knees bent at a 90-degree angle and your feet flat on the floor. Push back on your heels, straighten your legs, and pull your toes toward your shins.

Hold 2 to 3 second and repeat.

Maintain the arch in the lower back to target your hamstrings properly.

Glutes Stretch

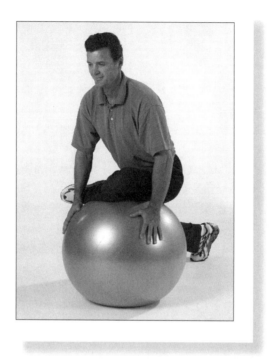

Place the side of your bent knee on top of the ball with the other leg extended behind you.

Place both hands on the ball in front of you (as you become more flexible, drop your hands toward the floor in front of you) while bringing your chest toward the bent knee. Roll the ball around to target different muscle fibers.

Stability Exercises

The following exercises force you to train in an unstable environment. These are great for golfers. In an unstable environment, the body's small but important joint stabilizers are engaged and strengthened. Strong joint stabilizers improve your ability to recruit larger, prime mover muscles, which results in an increase in power and strength. These exercises will also engage and strengthen the core, especially the small spinal muscles which can help you avoid lower back injuries. These will also help improve your balance, agility, and equilibrium.

Stability Exercises

Shoulder Stabilizer

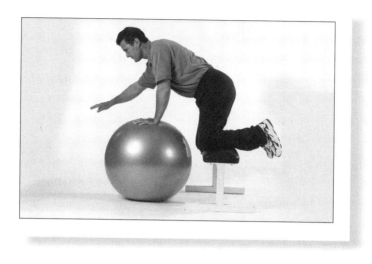

Place your hands on the bench directly under your shoulders. Your knees should be on the ball, hip width apart. Keep your spine aligned from the top of head to your tailbone and brace your abdominals. Remove one hand off ball. Maintain your squared shoulders and hip. Make small clockwise and counter clockwise circles with your supporting arm.

Static Bridge

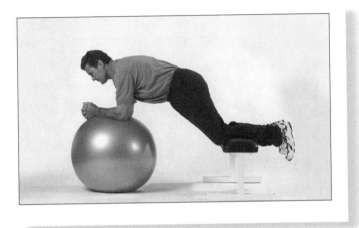

Place your knees on the bench and your elbows directly under your shoulders. Brace your abdominals and do not let your hips sag. Lift your hips slightly if you feel strain in your lower back.

A more advanced version has only the toes on the bench.

Stability Exercises

Knees on Ball Hands on Bench

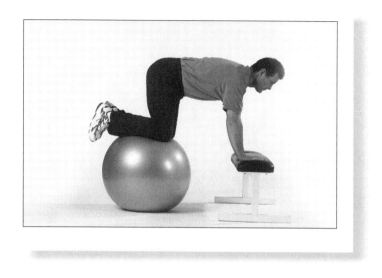

Place your knees on the ball and your hands on the bench. Bend your elbows slightly, and keep your head and neck in line with your spine. Brace your abdominals. Once you feel comfortable holding this position for 1 minute, attempt lifting one hand off of the bench.

Single Knee on Ball

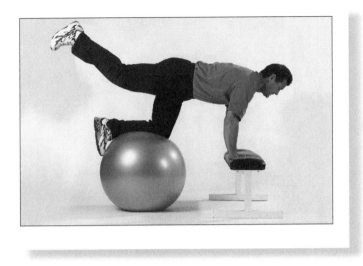

Place your hand on the bench with both your knees on the ball. Both your hips and trunk, and your arm and chest should be bent at a 90-degree angle. Keeping your head and neck in line with your spine, brace your abdominal and extend one leg behind you. Make sure to keep your hips square to the floor. Hold this position for 20 seconds. To increase the difficulty, increase by additional 20 second increments.

Stability Exercises

Perch with Wall

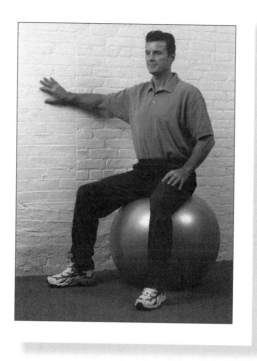

Place the ball next to a wall. Sit on the apex of the ball with your feet shoulder width apart. Your ears, shoulders, and hips should be in alignment. Once you feel confident, move the ball away from the wall.

Four-Point Perch

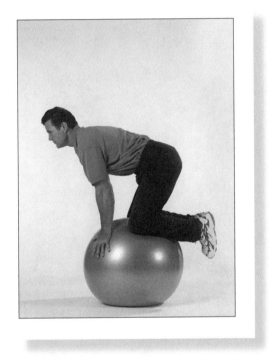

Stand in front of the ball. Place your hands on top of the ball and then gently allow your weight to roll you forward until your hands and knees are on the ball.

Three-Point Perch

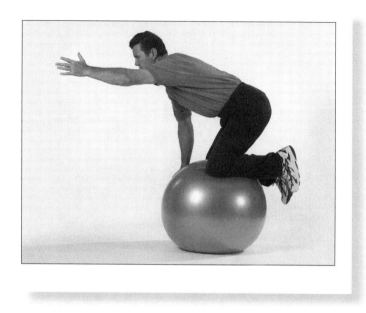

From the Four-Point Perch position, lift one hand off of the ball and extend the arm in front of you.

Two-Point Perch

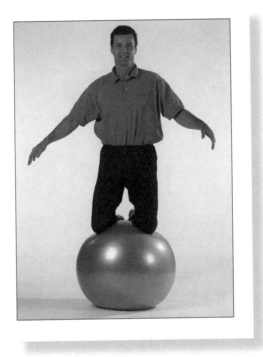

From the Three-Point Perch position, lift the remaining hand off of the ball. You must fully master the two-point stance position before attempting to apply weights in this position.

Upper Body Strength

Golfers need a strong upper body, shoulders, and arms to maintain complete control of the club head. If you are lacking in upper body strength and endurance, a variety of swing faults can be created. Golfers need to train for muscular endurance and strength—not for size. The *Golf Flex* program will target all the major muscle groups. These are the muscles most needed in the upper body to develop power during your swing.

Chest Press

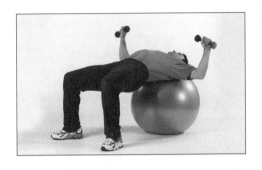

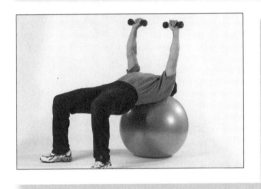

Start with a weight you feel comfortable with. Sit on the apex of the ball with your feet on the ground a bit wider than shoulder width apart. Hold the weights on your thighs, and slowly walk your feet forward until only your shoulders and head are resting on the ball. Lift the weights from your thigh to the starting positions–above the chest with your arms extended. Make sure your hips are elevated, keeping your knees, hips, and shoulders all in the same plane. Your knees should be directly over the ankles, with your lower and upper legs at a 90-degree angle. Lower the weight so the upper arms are parallel to your chest, then return to the starting position.

Be sure to keep your neck relaxed and position it on the ball so it maintains its natural curve. Also be sure the weights stay directly over the elbows during the full range of movement.

Push and Press

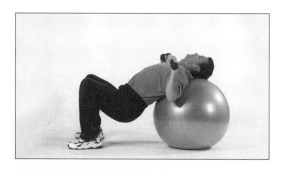

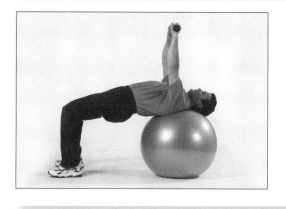

Start with a weight you feel comfortable lifting. Sit on the apex of the ball with your feet more than shoulder width apart. Slowly walk your feet forward, letting the ball roll slowly up your back until your head, neck, shoulders, and lower back are resting on the ball. Lower the dumbbells over your chest. As you press the dumbbells up over your chest, elevate your hips so that you're in the Tabletop position. As you lower the dumbbells, lower your hips again.

This engages the hips, legs, and chest, resembling a full-body pressing movement.

Upper Body Strength
Seated Lateral Raise

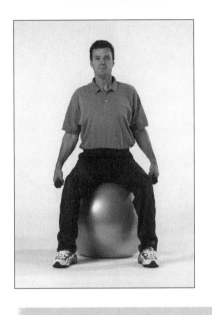 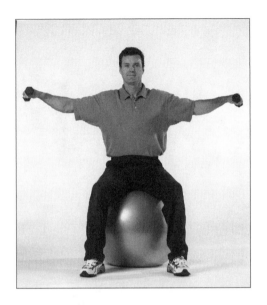

Sit on the apex of the ball. Maintain proper posture and keep your feet flat on the floor. Hold the dumbbells (palms down) by your sides, letting them rest on the side of the ball. Keeping your elbows bent slightly, slowly lift the dumbbells out to your sides and to shoulder height. Lower them, but don't let them rest on the ball again.

If you prefer, lift or press the weights over your head instead of raising them laterally. Do not allow the weights to rest on the ball while in the lowered position.

Two-Point Shoulder Press

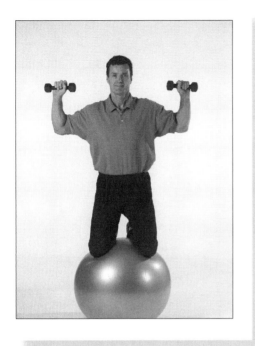
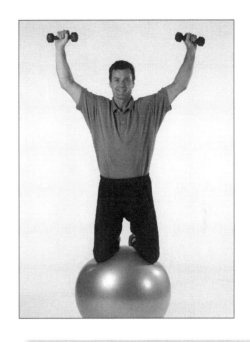

Hold the weights with your arms bent at 90-degrees. Press the weight over your head, and keep your belly drawn in tight.

This should be first done without any weight to establish a movement pattern.

Seated Anterior Raise

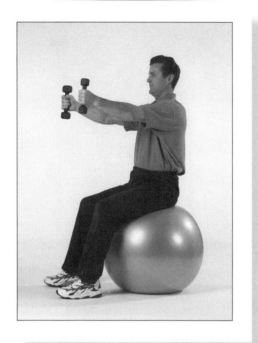 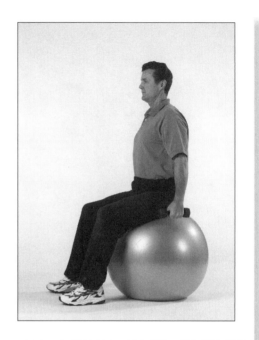

Sit on the apex of the ball. Maintain proper posture and keep your feet flat on the floor. Hold the dumbbells (palms facing inward) by your side, not letting them rest on the side of the ball. Lift the weights in front of you to shoulder height. Hold for a second before lowering the weights back to the starting position; repeat.

Maintaining proper shoulder position throughout the full range of motion is essential. Focus on keeping the shoulders down and in a seated position.

Two-Point Anterior Raise

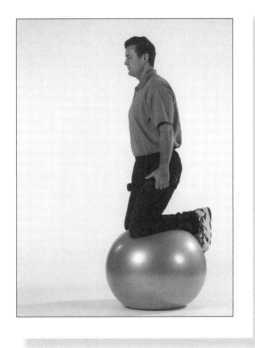 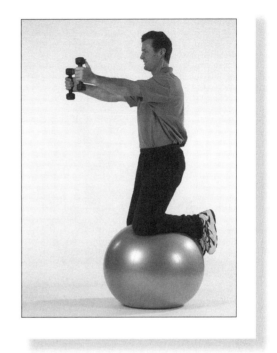

Kneel on the apex of the ball. Hold the dumbbells with your palms facing inward. Lift the weights in front of you to shoulder height. Hold for a second before lowering the weights back to the starting position. Repeat.

Seated Posterior Shoulder Press

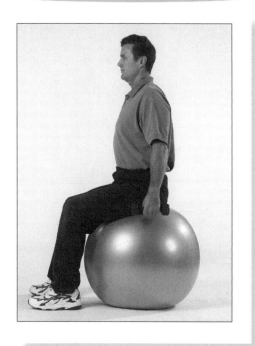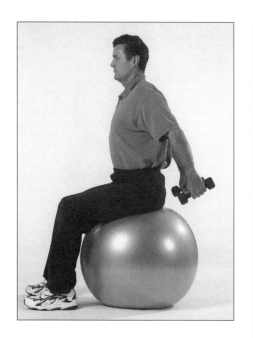

Sit on the ball with your feet hip distance apart. Keep your chest high and your shoulders back. Hold the weights by your side with your thumbs pointing forward. Press the weight backwards and squeeze your shoulder blades back at the same time.

Rear Delts

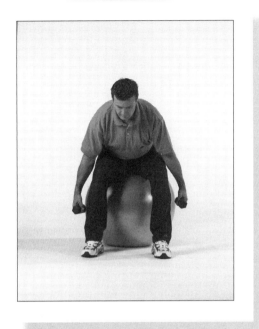 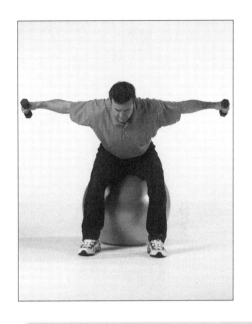

Sit on the apex of the ball. Maintain proper posture and keep your feet flat on the floor. Hold the dumbbells (palms facing inward) by your side. Bend at the waist so that your chest comes close to your knees and the weights are by your ankles. Lift the weights until they're parallel to the floor. Slowly lower them back to the starting position and repeat.

Maintain the curve in your lower back. It is essential to keep the belly button drawn in during this exercise.

Upper Body Strength
One-Arm Standing Row

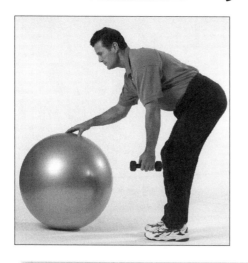 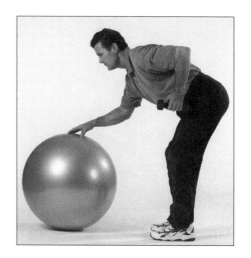

Place the ball in front of your right foot; place your right hand on the apex of the ball. Bend slightly at the knees. Keep your abdominals tucked in tightly. Hold a weight in your left hand. Let the weight hang with your arm fully extended; keep your shoulder blades back, in a seated position. Pull the weights backward, allowing your elbow to lead the way and sliding your arm along your waist. Repeat on the other side.

You can also train your trunk rotation by rotating at the waist when lifting the weight.

Two-Point Standing Row

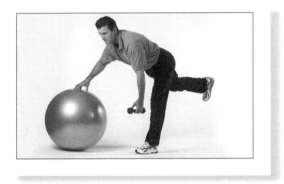

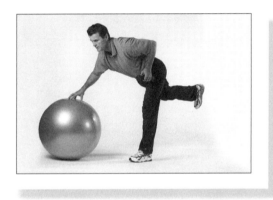

Place the ball in front of your right foot and place your right hand on the apex of the ball. Hold a weight in your left hand. Let the weight hang with your arm fully extended; keep your shoulder blades back, in a seated position. Elevate and extend your right leg behind you. Slightly bend your left leg and pull the weight backward, allowing your elbow to lead the way and sliding your arm along your waist. Repeat on the other side.

Upper Body Strength

Seated Biceps Curl

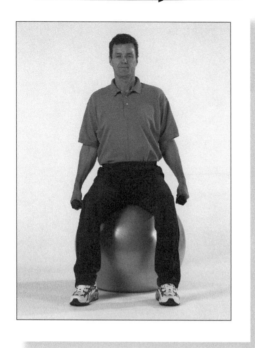 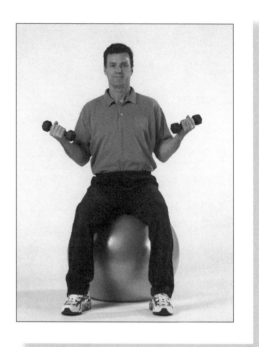

Start with a weight you feel comfortable lifting. Sit on the apex of the ball with your feet flat on the floor. Keep your chest high and your shoulders back. Let the weights hang by your sides, resting on the ball. Raise the weights with your palms facing your shoulders. Lower them, but don't let them rest on the ball again.

Try doing this with only one foot on the floor. This intensifies the exercise by incorporating your leg and trunk muscles.

Two-Point Biceps Curl

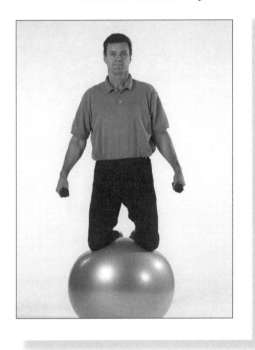 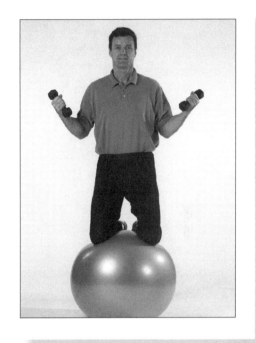

Approach the ball with the weights in your hands. Place your knees and hands on the ball and roll to a four-point stance. Lift yourself to a two-point stance. Maintain stable hips as you do biceps curls. Try curls working one arm at a time and then both arms at once.

You should not attempt this exercise until you're completely confident in your ability to maintain a two-point stance on the ball.

Seated Overhead Triceps Extension

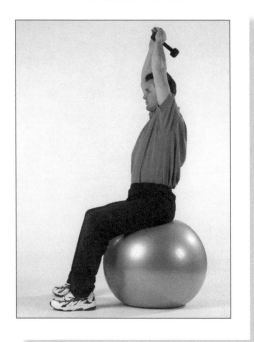 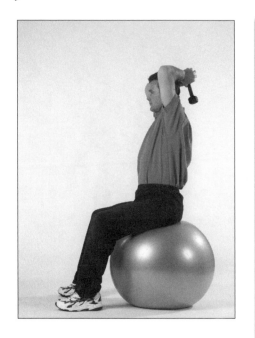

Start with a weight you feel comfortable lifting. Sit on the apex of the ball. Hold the dumbbell with both hands and place it over your head. Keeping the elbows parallel with each other, lower the weight behind your head with your forearms until your elbows are bent at a 90-degree angle. Press up with your forearms using the triceps muscle. Keep the elbows slightly bent in the uppermost position. Make sure that you keep your elbows close to your head at all times. Keep your upper arms fixed and elbows pointing up.

Tabletop Triceps Extension

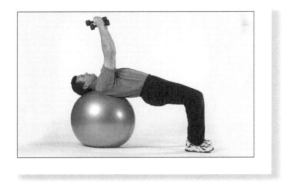

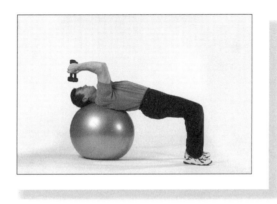

Start with a weight you feel comfortable lifting. Sit on the apex of the ball and roll down to the tabletop position. Once there, extend your arms over your chest. Bend your arm at the elbow, lowering the weights so that they're parallel to the floor.

Not only are you targeting your triceps, you engage your lower back, butt, hamstring, and core.

Lower Body Strength

Your power drive begins at its foundation: the legs. As the saying goes, "you can't shoot a cannon from a canoe." If you have a problem with posture, swaying, sliding, or weight shift, then you need to strengthen your lower body. The following exercises will develop your strength and stability, and will make your legs the building blocks for a powerful swing.

Split Leg Lunge

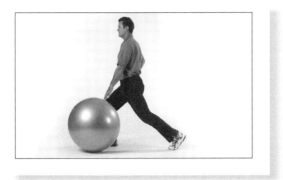

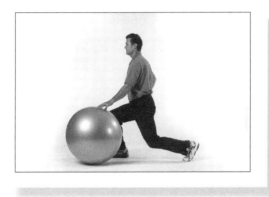

Standing with your feet hip distance apart, step forward with one leg. Place your fingertips on the ball for additional balance if needed. Lower the knee of your back leg towards the floor. Be very careful to not bounce your knee on the ground. The thigh of your forward leg should be parallel to the floor in its down position with your knee directly over the ankle. Do not bend forward at your waist. Keep your shoulders back and your chest high through the full range of motion.

Lunge and Roll

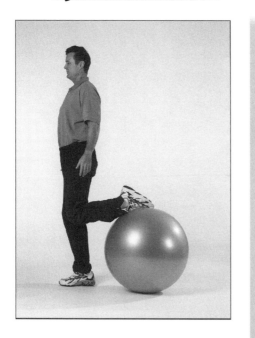 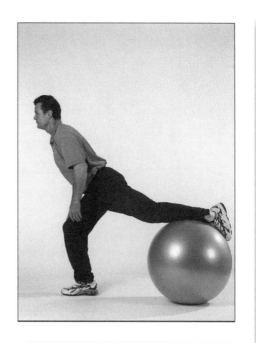

Stand with your feet shoulder width apart. Place your right instep on the ball behind you. Your knees should be parallel and the standing leg should be bent slightly. You can hold your hands out to the sides for more balance. Bend the standing leg and, at the same time, roll the ball backward with your foot. Lower yourself until the thigh of the lunging leg is almost parallel to the floor. As you straighten the front leg, roll the ball back to the original position.

Increasing the size of the ball will increase your free leg's hip flexors and flexibility.

Lower Body Strength
Wall Squat *good*

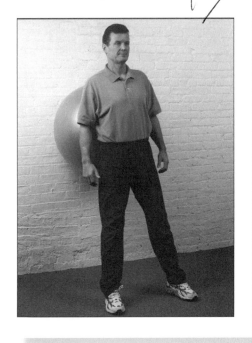
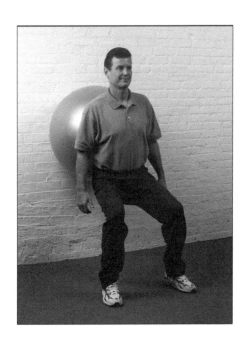

Stand in front of a wall with your feet at least shoulder width apart. Place the ball between your lower back and the wall. You should be far enough from the wall so that when you squat, your knees don't go beyond your toes. Keep your heels firmly on the ground. Slowly lower your butt to the level of your knees (the back of your thighs should be parallel to the floor) and then slowly return to the starting position.

For a more advanced version, hold weights in your hands as you do the exercise.

Single Leg Squat

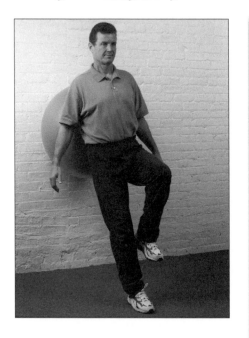 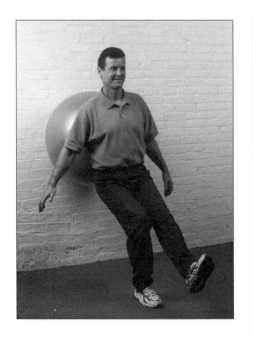

Stand in front of a wall with your feet at least shoulder width apart. Place the ball between your lower back and the wall. Lift one foot off the floor and lower yourself until the planted thigh is almost parallel to the floor. Slowly raise yourself again.

Be sure to line up your standing leg with the center of your body, not directly under the matching hip.

Lower Body Strength

Hamstring Curl

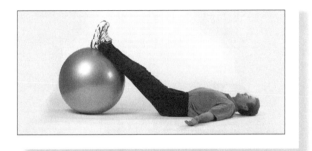

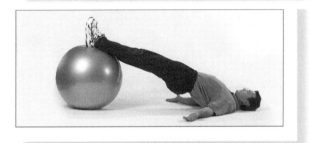

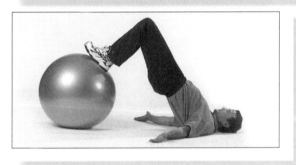

Lay face-up on the floor; place your ankles on top of the ball with your legs together. Keep your hips, shoulders, and head relaxed and on the floor. Extend your arms to your sides. Elevate your hips so that your ankles and shoulders are parallel, forming a straight diagonal line. Keeping your hips elevated, roll the ball in toward your butt. Roll the ball back out and then lower your hips to the floor. Move in a smooth, controlled manner: elevate the hips, curl in, curl out, lower the hips.

Avoid snapping your knee joint when you do this exercise; keep your knees soft.

Single Leg Curl

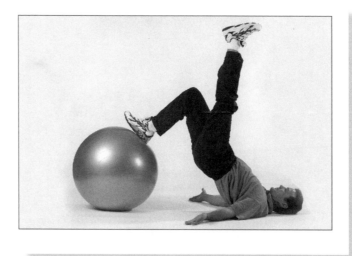

Lay face-up on the floor with your ankles on top of the ball and your legs together. Keep your hips, shoulders, and head relaxed and on the floor. Extend your arms (with palms down) at a 90-degree angle to your sides. Lift one leg straight up off the ball. With the other leg, roll the ball in toward your butt and then roll it back out and place the lifted leg back on the ball. Don't drop your hips back to the floor until you've completed the set; switch legs.

Lateral/One Knee on the Floor

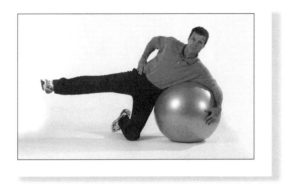

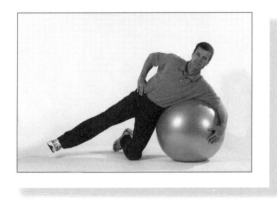

Kneel next to the ball and lean over it, with the side of your waist resting on the ball. Place one hand on the floor or the ball for stability. Keep the knee closest to the ball on the floor and extend your top leg. Lift your top leg in a controlled fashion. Avoid leaning forward or backward at your hip to make sure that your legs stay in line with each other.

45-Degree Inner Thigh Flex

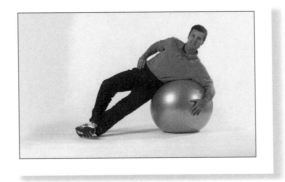

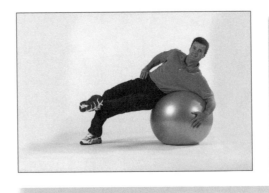

Lie on the ball on your hip with your legs stacked. Move the top leg onto the floor and in front of the bottom leg. Bend the bottom leg at a 90-degree angle. Raise the bottom leg a few inches off the floor and then lower it again.

Lower Body Strength

Tabletop Hip Extension

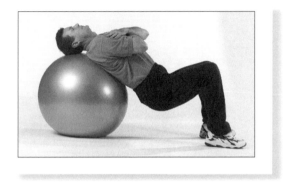

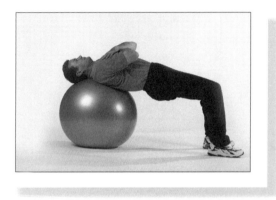

Sit on the apex of the ball with your feet shoulder width apart. Slowly walk your feet forward, letting the ball roll up your back until it reaches your shoulders. Your head and neck should be comfortably resting on the ball and your butt should be close to the floor. Press your hips up so that they are parallel to your knees and then lower your hips to the ball again.

Place a barbell plate on your hips to increase the intensity.

Single-Leg Hip Extension

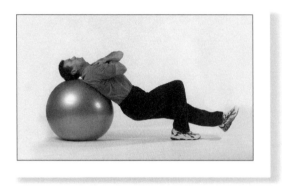

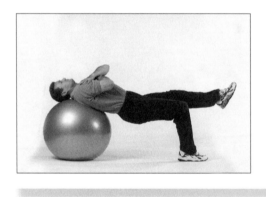

Sit on the apex of the ball with your feet shoulder width apart. Slowly walk your feet forward, letting the ball roll up your back until it reaches your shoulders. Your head and neck should be comfortably resting on the ball and your butt should be close to the floor. Lift one leg and extend it so that it's parallel to the floor. Stabilize yourself with the grounded foot. Keeping your hips square, press them up so that they are parallel to your knees. Slowly lower your hips back to the ball.

Core Strength

A strong core is essential for a consistent golf swing. Take a look at the mechanics: your hips stay relatively still, your shoulders rotate, and the burden to create the torque between the shoulders and hips rests with your abdominal muscles. If your abs are weak, you will never reach the full potential of your club head speed. A strong core will also keep stress off your lower back and help improve your posture.

Core Strength

Reverse Crunch

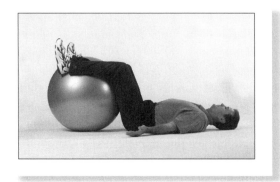

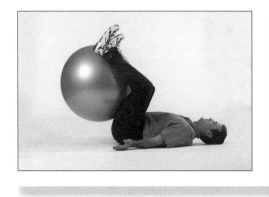

Lie on your back on the floor with your knees bent and legs on the ball. The ball should be wedged between your butt and calves. Lift the ball off the floor with your heels and draw your knees to your chest and then slowly return them to the floor.

If you feel any discomfort in your lower back, don't lower the ball all the way to the floor.

External Rotator

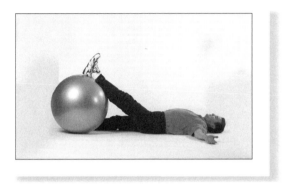

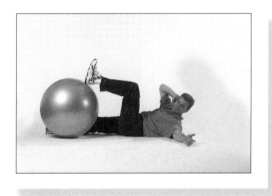

Lay on the floor with one leg extended. Place your other leg on the ball so that your knee is bent. With one hand behind your head, rotate your torso towards your bent knee. Focus on the lifting the back of your shoulder blade off of the floor and bringing the front of your shoulder towards your knee. Be careful to not reach towards your knee with the elbow. Keep your chin tucked in and support your head with your hand.

Core Strength

Internal Oblique

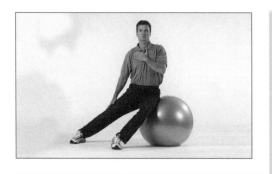

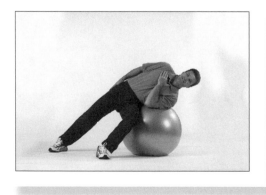

Place one buttock on the ball and bend your bottom leg to 90-degrees. Your top leg should be straight and you may place its foot against a wall for stability. Place your hands behind your head. Lower your shoulder toward the ball. Be careful to avoid turning or rotating your torso while following this movement.

The lateral crunch is a much needed and often ignored exercise. It targets the internal obliques on the side of the waist, which are major stabilizers of the lower back.

Back Extension

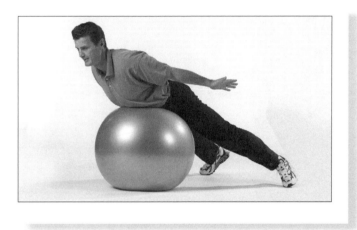

Lay with your hips on the ball and your feet wide apart behind you. Keep your knees off the floor. Place your hands, palms up, by your thighs. Lift your chest off the ball, rotate your palms toward the floor, and squeeze your shoulder blades together. Hold the up position for 3 seconds and then return to the starting position.

Core Strength

Crunch

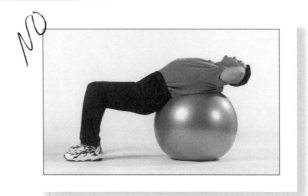

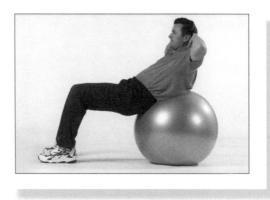

Sit on the apex of the ball with your feet shoulder width apart. Walk your feet forward until your lower back is firmly supported. Place your fingers by your temples; keep your elbows wide. Lower your upper back and shoulders onto the ball. Lift your upper back and shoulders off the ball to a roughly 45-degree angle. Keep your hips anchored so that you move over the ball, and the ball does not roll under you. Keep your tongue on the roof of your mouth to assist in engaging your deep neck flexors.

Doing crunches on the fitness ball increases the range of motion through which your abs must work.

Crunch with Rotation

No

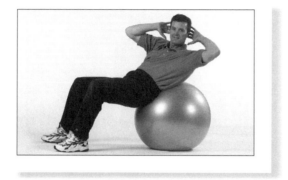

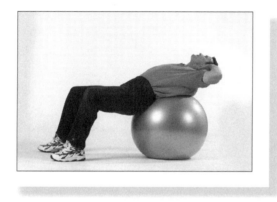

Sit on the apex of the ball with your feet shoulder width apart. Walk your feet forward until your lower back is firmly supported. Place your fingers by your temples; keep your elbows wide. Lower your upper back and shoulders onto the ball. Lift your upper back and shoulders off of the ball to a roughly 45-degree angle. As you do so, turn your torso to the left, then lower yourself. Repeat, switching sides.

This twist engages your obliques, which strengthens your shoulder-to-hip rotation.

Internal Oblique II

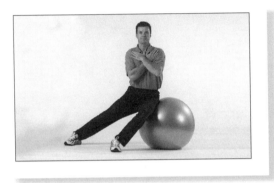

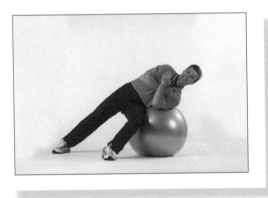

Place one buttock on the ball with your bottom leg bent at 90-degrees. Your top leg should be straight and its foot can be placed against a wall for stability. Cross your arm across your chest and laterally lower your torso so that your bottom shoulder touches the ball. Hold the torso as if there was a plane of glass in front of you. Avoid rotating.

The size of the ball will increase or decrease the intensity of this exercise. A larger ball gives you a smaller range of motion and is a good place for a beginner to start.

Advanced Back Extension

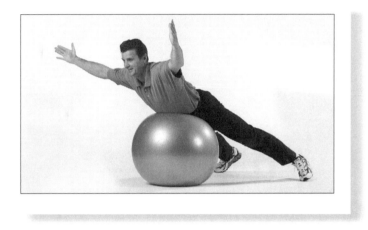

Lay with your hips on the ball and your feet wide apart behind you. Keep your knees off the floor. Place your hands, palms up, by your thighs. Lift your chest off the ball. As you do, squeeze your shoulder blades together and extend your arms in front of you. Hold the up most position for 3 seconds and then return to the starting position.

This requires a lot of back strength and stability.

Part VII:
30-Minute Exercise Ball Golf Workout

A beginner and an advanced version of an upper body and a lower body workout are provided in this section. You should always start your exercise ball workout with a good warm-up. Any of the cool down exercises may be added to the warm-up as long as they are performed in a dynamic fashion.

SIZING GUIDELINES FOR EXERCISE

YOUR HEIGHT	BALL SIZE
Under 5'2" (1.57m)	45 cm
5'3"–5'8" (1.60m-1.72m)	55 cm
5'9"–6'2" (1.75m-1.88m)	65 cm
Above 6'3" (1.90m)	75 cm

Beginner Upper Body Workout

Warm-up for Upper Body Workout
- Yes and Nos
- Shoulder Rolls
- Standing Rotations
- Supine Twist

Stability Upper Body
- **SHOULDER STABILIZER:** Hold for 1 to 3 minutes.
- **KNEES ON BALL:** Hands on Bench. Hold for 1 to 3 minutes.
- **SINGLE KNEE ON BALL:** Hold for 1 to 3 minutes.
- **TWO-POINT PERCH:** Hold for 1 to 3 minutes

BEGINNER UPPER BODY STRENGTH WORKOUT

EXERCISE	NO. OF SETS	NO. OF REPS	WEIGHT	TEMPO	RESTING INTERVAL
CHEST					
Chest Press	1-3	12-15	65-75%	2-1-2	<60 seconds
SHOULDERS					
Seated Lateral Raise	1-2	12-15	60-70%	2-1-2	<60 seconds
Anterior Raise	1-2	12-15	60-70%	2-1-2	<60 seconds
Seated Posterior Shoulder Press	1-2	12-15	60-70%	2-1-2	<60 seconds
BACK					
One Arm Standing Row	1-3	12-15	60-70	2-1-2	<60 seconds
ARMS					
Seated Biceps Curl	1-3	12-15	60-70%	2-1-2	<60 seconds
Seated Overhead Triceps Extension	1-3	12-15	60-70%	2-1-2	<60 seconds
CORE					
Reverse Crunches	1	20	Bodyweight	1-1-1	none
External Rotator	1	20	Bodyweight	1-1-1	none
Internal Oblique	1	20	Bodyweight	1-1-1	none
Back Extension	1	20	Bodyweight	1-1-1	none

Post Upper/Core Body Post Stretch/Mobilization
- Chest Stretch
- Shoulders Stretch
- Biceps Stretch
- Triceps Stretch
- Waist Stretch
- Back Stretch

Advanced Upper Body Workout

Warm-up for Upper Body Workout
- Yes and Nos
- Shoulder Rolls
- Standing Rotations
- Supine Twist

Stability Upper Body
- **SHOULDER STABILIZER:** Hold for 1 to 3 minutes.
- **KNEES ON BALL:** Hands on Bench. Hold for 1 to 3 minutes.
- **SINGLE KNEE ON BALL:** Hold for 1 to 3 minutes.
- **TWO-POINT PERCH:** Hold for 1 to 3 minutes

ADVANCED UPPER BODY STRENGTH WORKOUT

EXERCISE	NO. OF SETS	NO. OF REPS	WEIGHT	TEMPO	RESTING INTERVAL
CHEST					
Push and Press	2-3	12-15	70-80%	2-1-2	<45 seconds
SHOULDERS					
Two-Point Shoulder Press	1-2	10-12	60-70%	2-1-2	<45 seconds
Two-Point Anterior Raise	1-2	10-12	60-70%	2-1-2	<45 seconds
Rear Delts	1-2	10-12	60-70%	2-1-2	<45 seconds
BACK					
Two-Point Standing Row	2-3	10-12	70-80%	2-1-2	<45 seconds
ARMS					
Two-Point Biceps Curl	2-3	10-12	70-80%	2-1-2	<45 seconds
Tabletop Triceps Extension	2-3	10-12	70-80%	2-1-2	<45 seconds
CORE					
Reverse Crunches	1	20	Bodyweight	1-1-1	none
Crunches with Rotation	1	20	Bodyweight	1-1-1	none
Internal Oblique II	1	20	Bodyweight	1-1-1	none
Advanced Back Extension	1	20	Bodyweight	1-1-1	none

Post Upper/Core Body Post Stretch/Mobilization
- Chest Stretch
- Shoulders Stretch
- Biceps Stretch
- Triceps Stretch
- Waist Stretch
- Back Stretch

Beginner Lower Body Workout

Warm-up for Lower Body Workout
- Pelvic Tilts
- Hamstrings
- Quadriceps
- Supine Twist

Stability Lower Body
- **HIP EXTENSION:** Hold for 1 to 3 minutes.
- **KNEES ON BALL:** Hold for 1 to 3 minutes.
- **SINGLE KNEE ON BALL:** Hold for 1 to 3 minutes.
- **TWO-POINT PERCH:** Hold for 1 to 3 minutes

BEGINNER LOWER BODY STRENGTH WORKOUT					
EXERCISE	NO. OF SETS	NO. OF REPS	WEIGHT	TEMPO	RESTING INTERVAL
QUADS					
Split Leg Lunge	1-3	12-15	Bodyweight	3-1-3	<60 seconds
Wall Squat	1-3	12-15	Bodyweight	3-1-3	<60 seconds
HAMSTRINGS					
Hamstring Curl or Hip Extension	1-3	12-15	Bodyweight	3-1-3	<60 seconds
HIPS					
Lateral/1 Knee on Floor	1-3	12-15	Bodyweight	3-1-3	<60 seconds
GLUTES					
Tabletop Hip Extension	1-3	12-15	Bodyweight	3-1-3	<60 seconds

Post Lower Body Stretch
- Quadriceps Stretch
- Hamstrings and Calf Stretch
- Glutes Stretch

Advanced Lower Body Workout

Warm-up for Lower Body Workout
- Pelvic Tilts
- Hamstrings
- Quadriceps
- Supine Twist

Stability Lower Body
- **HIP EXTENSION:** Hold for 1 to 3 minutes.
- **KNEES ON BALL:** Hold for 1 to 3 minutes.
- **SINGLE KNEE ON BALL:** Hold for 1 to 3 minutes.
- **TWO-POINT PERCH:** Hold for 1 to 3 minutes

ADVANCED LOWER BODY STRENGTH WORKOUT					
EXERCISE	NO. OF SETS	NO. OF REPS	WEIGHT	TEMPO	RESTING INTERVAL
QUADS					
Split Leg Lunge	1-3	12-15	Bodyweight	3-1-3	<60 seconds
Wall Squat	1-3	12-15	Bodyweight	3-1-3	<60 seconds
HAMSTRINGS					
Hamstring Curl or Hip Extension	1-3	12-15	Bodyweight	3-1-3	<60 seconds
HIPS					
Lateral/1 Knee on Floor	1-3	12-15	Bodyweight	3-1-3	<60 seconds
GLUTES					
Tabletop Hip Extension	1-3	12-15	Bodyweight	3-1-3	<60 seconds

Post Lower Body Stretch
- Quadriceps Stretch
- Hamstrings and Calf Stretch
- Glutes Stretch

Golf Flex Strength Program

"What is tempo?" Tempo is the duration of each repetition of a particular exercise. It dictates the time in which your muscle is under weight bearing stimulus. For example, one rep of a bicep curl done at a 3:1:3 tempo would place the muscle under stimulas for 7 seconds. It would mean lifting the weight on a three count, holding it at the apex for a one count, and lowering at a three count.

"Why change tempo of an exercise?" Slow tempos of 3:1:3 are best for developing deep postural stabilizing muscles. Fast tempos of 1:0:1 are best for developing explosive power. Medium tempos of 2:1:2 are best for strength gains and maintenance of the primary muscle groups.

"How do I know how much weight or load to use?" Let your form be your guide. If you find yourself swinging the weights, and are not able to maintain good technique, the tempo, or properly stabilize yourself, you should lighten the load.

"How many sets are enough?" This depends of what condition you're in and if you've had resistance training before. Remember, we're training not straining. If you can only do one set, that's perfectly fine. Start with one and work yourself up to 3.

"How long will it take me to get stronger?" To see a real gain in strength it will take a commitment of 6 to 8 weeks. You may feel that the weight you are lifting is feeling lighter within a few weeks, but this is only because your body is becoming adapted to weight bearing exercises.

"Could I be creative with the exercise program?" If you're an experienced exerciser, sure. But remember that when you change one of the variables (set, reps, load, balance, or rest intervals) it often means decreasing one or more of the other variables.

"I really enjoy my program, why do I need to change it?" Your body will adapt to any given program over time, and when it does, you will stop seeing results. I know change is hard, but only by requiring your body to adapt to the demands of change in a program will result in a strength increase.

"Will my muscles get stiff and sore from strength training?" If you've had little experience with strength training, you may have some initial soreness. This can effect your swing. I suggest you begin a strength training program slowly and in the off or slow season.

"Won't bulking up ruin my swing?" Unless you're on some heavy steroids, you won't be getting Arnold-like muscles. The Golf Flex program will get you strong and stable—not bulky.

"Will I be totally exhausted after working out?" If you're exhausted after your workout you're working out too hard. The workout should feel challenging not impossible. You need to find the edge in the training. You should feel invigorated afterwards, not depleted.

For increasing strength in the stabilizing muscles and for beginners, start with:

Slow tempo of 3.3.3. Use a light load that you can complete 15 to 20 repetitions with

For general strength increase and for maintenance during golf season:

- Medium tempo of 2.1.2. Use a medium level of load that you can complete 10 to 12 repetitions with

For increasing power (strength and speed = power). Best pre or post golf season:

- Fast tempo 1.1. Use a heavy load in which you can perform 8 to 10 reps with

Strength training for golfers means more horse power!

Part VIII:
Conclusion

A Final Note

Golf Flex was developed out of necessity. As my golfing clients rolled in on Monday mornings complaining of muscle weakness and soreness after playing a couple of rounds of golf on the weekend, I encouraged them to stretch before and after every game.

The response I always got was, "Of course I stretch. Everyone stretches before the game. That's nothing new. Everyone knows the benefits of flexibility training and how it improves your game." So, if they were stretching, why were they always so banged up and sore? So I asked them how they stretched. The response was always the same. "Oh well, I . . . uh, you know, uh, . . . do some of these and then I swing the club around, and . . . uh, you know, loosen up."

It was pretty obvious that they didn't have a handle on what they were doing, and that they probably picked up most of what they did from what they saw other golfers doing on the course. Golfers know golf, not stretching. It was apparent they had no systemic approach to stretching that they could follow in a safe and effective way.

I developed *Golf Flex* so golfers could understand and perform stretches in a simple and clear manner. It is just as important for golfers to continue their stretching everyday to increase flexibility and range of motion in a progressive matter. *Golf Flex* not only improves your golf game, but also leads to increased body awareness and well-being. You can achieve results, so what are you waiting for? When it comes to stretching, there's never an excuse not to do something.

In health and fitness,
Paul Frediani

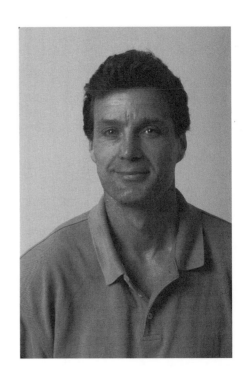

Meet the Author

Paul Frediani is one of America's leading fitness experts. He has been featured on national television and in magazines, including *Fitness*, *InStyle*, *Self*, and *Women's Wear Daily*. Certified by the American College of Sports Medicine and the American Council on Exercise, he is affiliated with Equinox Fitness Clubs in New York City, and is a C.H.E.K. level 1 practitioner. Paul's other fitness books include *Surf Flex*, *The Boot Camp Workout*, and the *PowerSculpt* series.